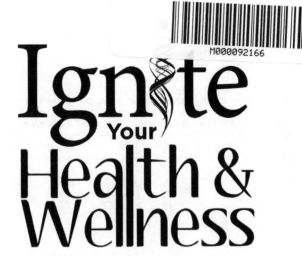

Ignite Your Health & Wellness

Thirty-six healing stories by those who have transformed their physical, mental and emotional lives.

FOREWORD BY

Marisa Peer

World Renowned Speaker, Rapid Transformational Therapy
Founder and Best-Selling Author.

INTRO BY

JB Owen

Founder of Ignite and JBO Global Inc.

PRESENTED BY

Alex Jarvis, Andrea Harrison, Ann Bridges, Annie Lebrun, Ariel Richards, Ben Ivanowski,
Brent McCord, Dr. Bryce Fleming, Cassandra Fox-Percival, Charlene Ray, Claes Nermark,
Dianna Delacoeur, Emily C. Ross, Felice Marano, Dr. Gregory Damato, Hilde Jahren,
Inga Ulmane, James McMillen, JB Owen, Katarina Amadora, Katelin Gregg,
LL Samantha Legassie, Marjan Tavakkolian, Maxime Šumberac, Mayssam Mounir,
M.D., Mystère Poème, Neil Cannon, Phyllis Roberto, Shannon Bliss, Tara Lehman,
Taylor Ribar, Teresa Irwin, Tina Lunde, Vera Mirna, Wendy Albrecht, Yaana Hauvroesh

Published by Ignite and printed by JBO Global Inc.

This book is dedicated to all who honor and respect their bodies, health and wellness. It is for those of us who are thinking bigger and beyond conventional medicine, and who believe that the spirit within has the power to heal and transform. It is for those who are looking inward versus outward, and finding the solution in the body itself. They are the ones blazing the trail using new techniques while maintaining the traditional ways of the past.

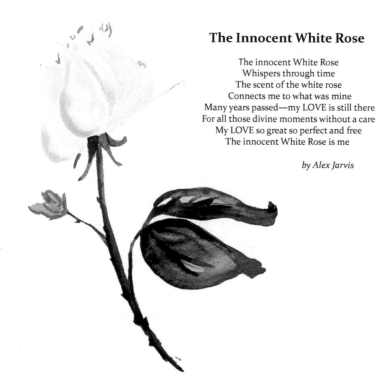

The Innocent White Rose

The innocent White Rose
Whispers through time
The scent of the white rose
Connects me to what was mine
Many years passed—my LOVE is still there
For all those divine moments without a care
My LOVE so great so perfect and free
The innocent White Rose is me

by Alex Jarvis

The rose is the highest vibrational flower. The white rose is a gesture of strong emotion and devotion having the meaning of spiritual love, charm and humility. The white rose at the front of this book is holding all the authors and readers in its highest vibration of pure LOVE.

AUTHOR TESTIMONIAL

"So honored to be part of this profound sharing of vulnerability, courage, triumph and healing wisdom. Blessed to have been invited to participate in this project! Still in awe of the powerful process of writing my story, and the loving professional support provided by the Ignite Team. Much appreciation! Ignite moments continue..."

— Yaana Hauvroesh - Canada

"The entire Ignite process happened very naturally. I had a powerful story to share – my truth to unveil and write out loud. Only a few words but such a massive change to offer in terms of cultural paradigm, pure hope for many people's lives. All it took me was to simply dream and dare enough to realize everything is possible. This is how Ignite came across my path at the right time – to help me manifest the writer I have always known I was. Thank you Ignite family!"

— Felice Marano - Italy

"As I laid out words on paper, I found my voice. I was stunned! Thank you, Ignite Team, for your support, your professional guidance and structure. I enjoyed every minute of it and had so much fun sharing this journey with other authors. A life-changing experience."

— Annie Lebrun - Germany

"I was doubting and scared but I signed up anyway. In two short months – carried by a wave of support and encouragement from the Ignite staff – I was gently set down on the shores of Success! I can hardly believe I did it! It was even fun and exciting! I recommend this experience for everyone. We all have a story to tell."

— LL Samantha Legassie - Canada

Ignite Your Health and Wellness Copyright © 2019 JBO Global Inc.

Publisher's Note: We are delighted to offer the sixth compilation book in the IGNITE series. Our mission is to produce inspiring, motivational and authentic real-life stories that will Ignite You in your life. Each book contains 35 unique stories told by 35 exceptional authors. They are of the highest caliber to offer engaging, profound and life-changing examples that will impact the reader. Our mandate is to build a conscious, positive and supportive community through our books, speaking events, writing workshops, ignite experiences, podcasts, immersions and a product marketplace. We welcome new authors onto our platform and new book ideas. Should you desire to be published and featured in an Ignite book, please apply at www.igniteyou.life/apply or reach out to us. suppport@igniteyou.life.

Published and printed by JBO Global Inc.

5569-47ᵗʰ Street Red Deer, Alberta

Canada, T4N 1S1 1-877-377-6115

Cover design by JB Owen

Book design by Dania Zafar

Designed in Canada, Printed in China

ISBN# 978-1-7923-0669-3

First edition: December 2019

Ordering Information: Quantity sales. Special discounts are available on quantity purchases by corporations, associations and others. For details, contact the publisher at the address above. Programs, products or services provided by the authors are found by contacting them directly. Resources named in the book are found in the resources pages at the back of the book.

Ignite Your Health & Wellness

INTRODUCTION BY
JB OWEN

Like many people who have seen the sun crest and set for quadruple decades, I found myself searching for more. I had run the gambit of great jobs and horrible ones. I had completed my school, constructed my dream home, had two kids and finalized more than one marriage. I had done a good job of living in the fast lane, pushing the stroller and chasing those unobtainable numbers on my bank statement. Life had blessed me in many ways and I had a plethora of memories plus a few battle scars to prove it. My existence had been traversing the same hamster wheel as most; work, obtain, then work some more to get more. I kept pushing and striving for the next funky gadget, the bigger horse-powered car and a nicer address.

In many ways, I thought I had it all. The material things others envied were in both my closet and garage. The 16,000 pictures on my phone said I had 'been places' and 'done stuff'… but at the end of the day, my heart and body were the ones dissatisfied in the mirror. The reflection I saw was limp and lackluster. The zeal I was supposed to feel from all my accomplishments was like a wet paper napkin after a holiday meal, drenched in too much overindulgence to be useful. I was taxed out physically and emotionally from wanting it all and my health began to deteriorate.

I ignored my constant constipation, mood swings and horrible menstrual cramps. If my stomach became bloated, I told myself it was because of something I ate. If my feet itched so much in the night it stopped me from sleeping, it was because of the detergent I was using. When my hands broke out in a rash,

I convinced myself it was due to an overindulgence of sun. Any little ailment I experienced I'd brush off and accuse some external factor as the culprit. I didn't connect the dots that it was my body's way of giving me a message, and that discomfort and unease were big indicators I should be paying attention to.

Instead, I kept doing what I had always done; I ignored it. I brushed off how I was feeling and buried it under a litany of practical excuses. I was a master at justifying a pang in my temple as my pillow's fault and uncontrollable sneezing fits due to something in the air. Never once did I think those things were my body's way of screaming for me to pay attention. To stop eating food that was irritating my stomach, to get up from my desk after countless hours and consume some much-needed water. I didn't see the connection between the odd outbreaks my body was exhibiting and the unsettled emotions that I was bottling up inside.

Until I met the lovely Marisa Peer, an extraordinary woman who gracefully approached me one afternoon at a conference we were attending. She was delightful to talk to and fabulously interesting. An instant friendship began and I happily saw Marisa countless times after that, talking about business ideas, upcoming travel, my children and the projects we were both working on.

When I saw Marisa on stage speaking a few years later, I truly witnessed all that lay beneath her adoring charm and brilliant mind. Her positive approach and common-sense attitude toward eliminating self-manifested problems was intriguing. She spoke in such an eloquent and sensible way, you couldn't help but see the logic behind it. Her concepts on the power of the mind, the words you use and the things you think... got me thinking! What we say really matters. How we command our thoughts has an impact and the language we use becomes the language our body responds to.

Marisa always took the time to listen to my points of view and kindly gave me alternative ones to ponder. She had a way of opening up my mind to brighter ideas and dissolving my opinions in ways that seemed practical and doable.

One day while having lunch in the glistening sun on the island of Ibiza, Spain, Marisa gave me some advice that shook the foundation of my core. I was bringing her up to speed on the latest developments in my life while I was scratching the back of my hands. She asked me why I was doing that and I told her I always get a rash on my hands when I spend too much time in the sun. "Always?" she questioned.

"Yes," I told her. It happens whenever I am overdoing it and exposed to too much UV.

"Why are we sitting in the sun then?" she asked curiously.

It was such a simple question, but her tone and demeanor of genuine inquisitive introspection broke through the layers of my token response and I stopped, mouth wide open, unable to answer. She looked at me quizzically without any judgment and waited for me to reply. I paused, struggling to find my words. It was as if my mind went blank and the autopilot excuses I usually made were down in an unattainable well of illogical reasoning. Marisa's inquiry reached a deeper part of me that began searching for the REAL answers. All the excuses I had made in the past were fragmented in my mind and I couldn't find words to formulate the truth. For the first time since I started having that problem, I actually asked myself… "Why *am* I sitting in the sun? Why, if my hands are already irritated, am I still exposing them to more of the thing I believe is the cause?"

As we went on with our meal, my mind was reeling inside. Marisa had cracked open a door and a flood of questions poured in. Why did I continue to do what was contributing to my ailment? Why was I not honoring my body? What was the REAL reason my hands would break out? Why had I gone most of my life just accepting it, not doing something to preempt it or even to stop adding to it when it happened? All these questions began swirling in my head and I started asking my body for the answers, sitting with myself and going within to search out both the reason and the solution. I wanted to uncover the true cause and do something to fix it. I was no longer willing to just ignore the symptoms and passively endure them. This lead me down a path of more internal exploration and personal growth.

Which lead me right back to Marisa.

Sitting at a conference in Costa Rica I had the pleasure of undergoing one of Marisa's RTT sessions. She took us back to the origin point of many of our issues and aliments. Her decisive therapy technique and hypnotherapeutic modality went right to the internal root of the cause and repaired it. It was a transformative moment indeed! Since then, I have enjoyed many more of Maria's life-changing sessions. Her powerful process is both easy and impactful. Marisa truly helps you heal from within and recode your thinking to be self-affirming and successful. She instills a new mindset that dissolves the underlying issues and teaches you how to fill your thinking with the thoughts that will allow you to have the life you desire.

Marisa truly is a healer from the heart and her mission to help others is apparent in everything she does. She is an example of using your thoughts and words to empower and propel you to live your ultimate dreams. I love her dearly and I know you will too.

"When you can collaborate with your mind and tell it what you want, you will get what you want." Marisa Peer

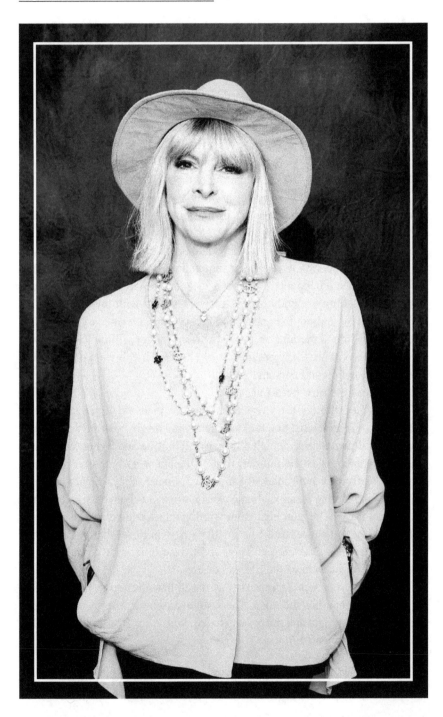

FOREWORD BY
MARISA PEER

"Nothing gives me more fulfillment than
helping people live a healthy and happy life."

As an international therapist and Founder of Rapid Transformational Therapy™ (RTT™), I have spent over thirty years studying the mind, applying leading principles with thousands of clients who have achieved the most phenomenal results. Just like the authors in this book, I love sharing what I have learned, so that you can benefit from it in your life.

As you read this book and see some of the remarkable stories and challenges that people have overcome, you will know that the human body and mind is incredibly powerful and this book proves just what is possible in the area of optimum health and total wellness.

The person who has the most powerful potential to dictate your health, to make you healthy and to keep you healthy is not a doctor, not a drug, not a pill, not a psychologist, it's you.

You have the most incredible power to decide what kind of health you want to have and to keep that health for a long, long time. Like many people, I didn't know this when I was growing up; I had the same belief that most of us have. If you're ill, go to a doctor, they'll give you some medication and you get better. I did that for years.

One day, I heard a doctor say to me, "You can never have children, you're infertile, you can't get pregnant and you can't carry a baby to full term." I heard this clear voice in my head say, "Don't let that in." I really listened to that voice and I remember saying to the doctor, "I'm going to leave now, because I'm not going to let that in." and I left his office.

I decided not to let that in and many years later I got pregnant despite being told that it was physically impossible for me. When I got pregnant, I heard many other doctor's voices saying, "You won't be able to carry this baby to full term; this baby could have all kinds of things wrong with it." and I didn't let those voices in either. In fact, I had a perfect, healthy, gorgeous baby.

Many years later I heard a doctor's voice saying something I never thought I would hear. He said, "You have cancer." I was really shocked because I was healthy and I believed in the power of the mind. I asked him a question, "Will I get it again?" This doctor did something very odd. He knocked on the table with his fist and said, "Well, the cancer has your address, it knows where you live and it will probably come back." That was a huge sign for me not to let that in and actually, without wanting to sound glib, I sailed through cancer. It was just a blip. I felt amazing all the way through it and I got completely better very quickly. I've always been on path and I would love you to take that same path, where you take control of your own health. Don't give that power to someone else.

The truth is that you have phenomenal power to become well and stay well. That doesn't mean you'll never get ill, but you have amazing powers to heal your own illnesses. I created my own technique for doing this and I now teach people Rapid Transformational Therapy™ (RTT™), to treat all kinds of physical illnesses, mental illnesses, and emotional issues. I don't just treat the symptoms, I always look at what is really going on. I am a great believer that we can't always fix what we don't understand.

So many of the illnesses and ailments that I treat are not caused by a diseased organ at all, but what I call diseased thinking. I work with many doctors and hospitals who tell me that many people going to the Emergency Room have real physical symptoms, real traumas, real headaches, rashes, and sickness, but it's not caused by a diseased organ, it's caused by diseased thinking. Once you understand that, then you'll be able to think "Okay, well if I have the power to make myself ill, I certainly have the power to make myself better."

We already know that the mind can create physical symptoms. If we are embarrassed, we blush. If we are upset, we cry. If we are nervous, we shake. Your mind is capable of creating all kinds of physical symptoms, I think the mind can create the symptoms of almost any illness in the world. However, it can also get rid of those symptoms and work to overcome illness. During my 33 years as a therapist, I've worked with people with migraines, infertility, stuttering, inflammation, and every kind of skin disorder. I've had phenomenal success at helping them overcome their issues and I now have a deep understanding of the cause of illnesses, even depression.

To understand yourself so that you can have radiant, phenomenal health and a long healthy life, you need to understand what I call The Rules of Your Mind. Your mind's main job is to keep you alive and essentially your mind will always do what it thinks is in your best interest. Your mind's number one job is not to make you happy, it's to keep you alive on the planet. Our mind is often creating things that it believes are protecting us. You see, your mind is hardwired to move you away from pain and towards pleasure.

If your mind thinks that something is causing you pain, it will do everything in its power to make sure that you never have to go through that pain again. Many people say things like "If another relationship ends, I'll die" or "This stress is killing me." "My kid/partner/boss is driving me crazy." They are throwaway words, of course we don't mean them, but our mind takes everything we say literally. It believes what we tell it. Our words shape our reality and when our reality doesn't please us, then we have to change the words that shape it. The way that you feel about everything is down to the pictures you make in your head and the words you say to yourself.

I learned this when I worked with infertile women, they were my best teachers. Once I made the decision to get pregnant and have the perfect baby, despite being told that I couldn't, I realized I could help so many other women. Working with women with unexplained infertility and secondary infertility was such an eye opener for me. They would say things like "yeah I don't know why I can't get pregnant, but I remember when I was 15 thinking I was pregnant being absolutely terrified and praying that I wasn't..." Or, "When I had my first baby, I said I could never go through that again and now I've got secondary infertility." These things are just little lessons for us to understand that our mind eavesdrops on everything that we say, it believes everything we say and it works to make that real.

Every word you say, every thought you think is a blueprint that your mind and body must work to make real. The strongest force in all of us is that we must act in a way that matches our thinking and our mind really doesn't care if what we tell it is good or bad, right or wrong, healthy or unhealthy. It simply believes it. That's why it's so important not to say things like "I always... get sinus headaches in the winter, I always... get a bad back when I'm stressed,

I always… get food poisoning when I go on holiday." When you say those things, without even knowing it, you're making it real.

It's so easy to change your words from "I have a weak immune system, I have terrible digestion, I always get sick," to "I have a phenomenal immune system, I have great digestion, I'm strong and healthy." Choose your words carefully. You make your beliefs and then your beliefs make you, and then you find proof that your beliefs are real. Make your beliefs about your health amazing, positive and powerful.

Enjoy this collection of some of the best real life stories from 36 outstanding individuals and health care practitioners, sharing their power quotes, intentions, ignite stories and action steps. Their goal, like mine, is to inspire you to live the most optimum life in both your health and your wellness. To do what you love is to have purpose, to share that with others is to have meaning. Use the stories here in this wonderful book to help you adopt better beliefs. When you see what these writers have done to take back their health you can use their stories and become empowered to do the same.

I support you in stepping into your greatest health and invite you to also use RTT. To find out more, please go to www.marisapeer.com or www.rapidtransformationaltherapy.com

PREFACE

The Health Nirvana

Many have said, "When we have our health, we have everything." A life of good health and optimum wellness is becoming the new million-dollar dream. What was once a race for materialistic gain has now become a desire for clean origins, a great physique and infinite longevity. A holistic lifestyle has moved to the forefront of the idyllic dream. To live long and healthy, able to age gracefully while doing lots of amazing things is the vision of the future that many of us have. To expire from age versus illness is the end goal on the minds of those seeking true happiness. The collective shift is moving toward success in our health, not our bank accounts.

In the upcoming pages of this book, you are going to read many stories of men and women living in the new 'health nirvana.' These individuals have stepped into the realm where living in their ideal health IS the foundation of their dream. You will read how they have moved away from conventional processes and producers to find a better, more meaningful life while optimizing their personal health. Some are doctors, others are not. Many are practitioners, health professionals and coaches who have stepped into healing the body in new, innovative ways. Others are regular people whose health has taken them on a road to awareness. Where their body's own system needed to wake them up and have them pay attention. These are the accounts of how their ailment or health crisis was a catalyst for a new style of living.

All of the authors in the book have shifted their lives from being told how to heal to healing from within. They have traversed the journey toward finding out what it means to be healthy and overcome the dis-ease and dis-comfort that were mere words written on a health form or hospital record. Their stories are the ones where the process was not to get to a final diagnosis but instead to feel a different way. To rid themselves of any illness using unconventional methods. To be in the driver's seat of their problem, not led around by someone who went to school and wore a white-colored lab coat.

You are about to embark on stories that clearly show healing is possible. That alternative ideas and alternate modalities have merit. That unique options and radical thinking can have transformative results. That by deeply getting involved in every aspect of their healing, the authors were able to achieve just that: a healthier existence.

All of the stories in this book have one common denominator: our health is our own. Each individual needs to listen to their body, learn about it, investigate its needs, try new things and absolutely believe in the messages it delivers. These authors show how the state of the body is a reflection of the state of the mind. And how the symbiotic connection between the two is paramount. The body responds to what the mind perceives and the mind is the epicenter of the health we feel.

Healing You

Throughout this book, you will read numerous stories of people healing and transforming their health. Many defy what we know about modern medicine and question the very conditioning of relying on an outside source to heal an internal issue. All the stories are shared to awaken you in your own healing endeavor. To empower and inspire you to find the modalities that are right for you. These are the stories designed to Ignite the most inner part of you: that deep connection you have with the body you live in and the mind that you live from.

This book is filled with many examples of overcoming physical issues and finding other means by which to heal and feel healthy. The stories run the gambit of health concerns from stress and overexertion to depression and mental health. Some authors have spoken about conditions such as alopecia, eczema and inflamed bowels. Others have tracked improvements in cancer, epilepsy, multiple sclerosis and chronic back pain. All have shared the ways that they found to harness their dis-ease and manage it better. To live richer and fuller lives despite a diagnosis. To be happier and healthier by embracing and knowing their condition intimately, and the ways to extricate it from their lives.

Ignite Your Health and Wellness was born from the idea that what we have been taught over the years is not the only form of healing. That the 'system' that governs pain management and 'dis'-ease control is often limited by the pharmaceutical solutions available on a prescription pad. Often, how the body reacts, feels, responds and processes is overlooked and the patient becomes a series of hypotheses and mysteries to figure out.

The stories you are about to read are the true accounts of 36 individuals looking beyond any manufacturer's parameters to find other opportunities and new possibilities in their entire holistic health. Each one relates their own personal journey and specific experience. They are not offering a medical solution or professional advice, they are simply sharing that other options gave them a profoundly different outcome.

My wish is that when you read through these stories, you are deeply transformed by the many examples of unique healing journeys that lead to better, more exquisite health. I hope that your mind opens and your self-awareness awakens to how powerful you are on your own healing path. That you feel the possibilities and potential that each one of the authors shares, and the supportive intentions behind their sharing. All the authors wrote their stories so that you may relate to the healing process within it. Every chapter was written with the hope of empowering you to be our own advocate on your personal quest to feeling amazing. That you discover and design your magnificent life with your health at the center of it.

As you turn the upcoming pages, you will find each story begins with a *Power Quote*. It is like a mantra or an inner activating phrase. Every individual should have one. It is a statement that pushes you to do even more and makes you think a little deeper. It is what your bumper sticker would say, or what you'd write on your office wall. Power quotes are words that you might repeat over and over when you need an extra boost, or when the tears are flowing from both life's hardships and rewards. Each Power Quote is designed to remind you of what you have inside, what you prefer to feel and how you can find a happier version of you.

Next, you will read each author's *Intention*. These are the insights and ideas they wish to inspire in you. They are personal messages filled with meaning and purpose. The authors want to IGNITE You to begin living your most extraordinary life and they share what they hope their insights will do for you. Their intentions set the tone for their message and are designed to both awaken and elevate your thinking.

Then, their inspiring *Story* follows. It is an honest sharing by each author as they explain how they found the answers to some difficult and lingering questions. These are their genuine accounts of consciously awakening to the *Ignite* moment that instigated a beautiful journey towards restoring their health. We all have *Ignite* moments in our lives that change us, define us and set us on a new path or trajectory. These stories are those moments, told in the most vulnerable and heart-felt way. They show that we all have *life-changing* moments that not only impact us but ultimately transform us.

Once you have finished their stories, you will find a list of *Ignite Action Steps*. These are the tangible things they did to heal and redefine themselves. Each author shares easy-to-do, practical tips for you to try and implement immediately. They are the processes and practices that worked in their lives. Each one is different and unique, just like you, and is proven to yield magnificent results when done consistently.

We all know actions speak louder than words; never is that more important than with your physical health. Action IS the key. To move the needle forward in your wellness, we encourage you to try one action step each day and do it consecutively for 30 days. We have offered you many different action steps to try, so find the one that feels fitting for you. Each one is potentially the step that could change your life forever. Start with the one that resonates the most and follow through to see significant and wonderful change throughout your life.

The most important thing we all want for you is for something you read to change you. For one of our stories to have a profound impact and push you in a new direction. For something to resonate and hit you so strongly, you *have* to take action. This is the most important thing. That one of our suggestions pushes you into a new conscious realization in your own life and you feel ready to transform. Ready to LIVE FULL OUT! You get to decide how to live and how to feel; no one else is in charge of that. Make the most of that power. Let these stories remind you that you can do anything, be anything and accomplish anything you choose. You can joyfully move forward and find your bliss. Your life can be absolutely wonderful on every level; you just have to decide first and then move consciously forward in that direction.

Heal from the Heart

We know that many people read compilation books to be inspired. If you feel that your story is still unfolding or you're trying to figure it out, we are with you. We have all been through difficulties and go through them numerous times in our lives. Our stories show our transformation in spite of all that. We still have issues, like everyone else; we have just learned and studied more to push ourselves and go forward. The learning behind all of us is now behind you too. We support you unconditionally and are cheering you on as you uncover your own healthy lifestyle. We extend our hands should you need a bit of support, some advice or a friend to confide in. We offer our services should you ever want to reach out because something we said resonated with you or what we shared was exactly what you needed to hear. Please know we are all accessible and eager to connect, so please feel free to find us. We are happy to support you as you undergo your own healing exploration.

Everyone needs support to rise and flourish. We all need to help each other in as many ways as we can. For everyone in this world to feel healthy, some must first forge the path. On your road to healing, you will be challenged and confronted; but if you are true to your inner knowing, those challenges will be met with the purest results. In your desire to regain your health, follow your heart and overcome any obstacles along the way. Seek out all that you need so you can make powerful decisions about your life. Focus on you, your needs, feelings and healthiest desires. Accentuate your gifts and shine your light. Give all you can to your holistic happiness because you are worth it!

I am ignited by the idea of you turning the next page and reading the many stories of health and wellness. I am excited that you are about to find out how another person stepped into the very essence of their healthiest life. Some may be filled with pain and suffering. Others might be riddled with disappointment or even tragedy. All show a determination and perseverance in the steps they needed to take to get where they needed to be. Their stories are a guide to the unlimited possibilities that are before you in your life. Be motivated by what they have shared and then decide to go out and do the same. Feel revitalized to venture forth in your life with a smile beaming on your face. Move and groove with excitement. Reclaim your health! That's the true magic in life. That's what makes it wonderful and worth living.

The stories you are about to embark on are all our stories. They supersede race, culture, age and even gender. They are the human story, the experience of being a Being on this earth. They touch at the very heart of belonging, connecting and sharing. They are raw, real and unrestricted… that's what makes them so amazingly engaging. They cut through all the 'stuff' we want people to see and shine a light directly on the heart of who we were born to be. Ignite was created to ignite others and impact humanity. Our mandate is to do more, share more and spread a conscious positive message to as many people as possible. We believe in the human connection. We believe that power comes from being heard, being seen and belonging to something greater than one's self.

We invite you to Ignite others. To let your story be heard, share your experiences and find your voice. We pride ourselves in bringing people together, offering a solution, giving back and doing something good for the planet. That is the mission and purpose behind IGNITE. There is power when one person touches the heart of another and a spark begins. Be it inspiration, love, support, encouragement, compassion or belief, we choose to Ignite it all. Each of us deserves to be Ignited and we hope these stories Ignite you.

May you have many ignite moments that transform your life into the amazing person you were meant to be. — JB Owen

Please know that every word written in this book, every letter in these pages, has been meticulously crafted with fondness, encouragement and a clarity not just to inspire you but to transform you. Many people in this book stepped up to share their stories for the very first time. They courageously revealed the many layers of themselves and exposed their weaknesses as few do. Additionally, they spoke authentically from the heart and wrote what was true for them. We could have taken their stories and aimed for perfection, following every editing rule; but instead, we chose to leave their unique and honest voices intact. We overlooked exactness to foster individual expression. These are their words, their sentiments, their explanations. We let their personalities shine in their writing so you would get the true sense of who each of them is completely. That is what makes IGNITE so unique. Authors serving others, stories igniting humanity. No filters. No desire for perfection. Just realness between us and you.

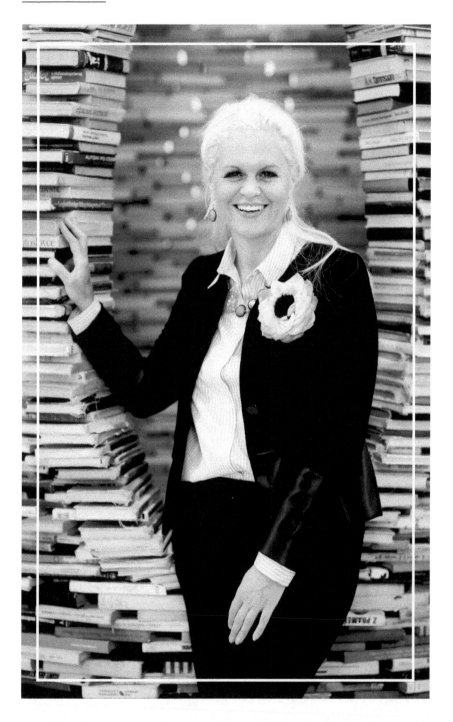

JB OWEN

"Words have life in them. If you say them, you become them."

Please say out loud… *I will gain great learning from this story and transform my life in a positive way.* **You have just activated that truth and set in motion a multitude of circumstances that will conspire to make it happen. Words have power. You can transform and materialize simply by speaking them. They have a life force all their own. Each one carries with it a directive to execute and a purpose to perform. Each of us experience and become exactly the words we use and the things we say out loud.**

WORD FORCE ENERGY

The word 'workaholic' was often spoken by my family. It was used to describe my parents in both a positive and prideful way. My parents were entrepreneurs, the best kind of workaholics, individuals determined to put in insurmountable hours and do over and above what the average worker would do. They wanted to *achieve* MORE, *do* MORE, and *be* MORE, and their workaholism became a normal component of my everyday life.

I grew up with a similar sense of pride. My parents were accomplishing things my friends' parents were not... and we had the stuff to show for it: swimming pool in the backyard, a Cadillac in the garage, a small Cessna 5-seater plane at the local airfield and a 40ft boat moored on the coast. Sometimes our family would fly 1400 kilometers just to spend the weekend on the boat. It was a privileged life, that came at a cost.

As a child, I learned that working was like breathing. It was mandatory. My mother often said, "You're just a waste of skin if you're not working," — a set of words I took too literally as a child. I started my first business when I was nine. I lied about my age and began working at 14. By 16, I had two jobs and I went on to spend the next two decades working insatiably at everything from cruise ship director to fashion designer to set supervisor in the film and television industry. At the height of my career, I was working 90 hours a week. When my paycheck arrived every two weeks, I'd rip open the envelope not to see the amount, but to make sure I had capped 180 hours. 181.7 was great and 183.9 was a celebration, anything less felt like a failure, I would be angry with myself for slacking off. If ever there was a bar, I made sure to supersede it. That meant longer hours and extra days, always the first to arrive and last to leave. I was the walking, talking, over-achieving poster-girl of a self-pro-claimed workaholic.

But like any addiction, my work habits had a dark side: enormous stress, debilitating sleep patterns, perpetual brain fog and erratic food consumption to help manage the highs and lows. It was like a thousand venomous coils squeez-ing the life out of me as I blatantly consumed my own tail. Just when I'd get a breath of reprieve, I'd step back in, entwining myself in another project, a heavier workload. I was suffocated by my own devices and engulfed in the frenzy of aspiring to do MORE.

Like all good addicts, the day came when I overdosed on my vice of choice. I was finishing up a 93-hour week, trudging outdoors in the pouring rain, moving something by myself that technically needed two people to move. I was hoisting a tremendous weight and turning at the same time when I heard a gaseous pop. My legs suddenly lost all sensation and I felt as if my bottom half had turned to sand, dissipating slowly into a dusty pile beneath me. Like a balloon fizzling to the ground, I withered, losing my balance and falling backward with the full weight of the object falling upon me. I laid there stunned, raindrops plunking down on my face and my embarrassment flaring. I pushed the weight off of me and rolled onto my side to get up. But I couldn't. My lower half was like a cocoon encased in cement. My body was going into shock. Lying in a puddle unable to move, hands shaking uncontrollably, I reluctantly called out for help.

That was the beginning of my recovery from my addiction. It marked the day my rehab began. I was admitted into the hospital with a torn disc in my spine and was immediately put into a steel pelvic brace and immobilized by traction. Everything I knew about myself felt pinched in a terrifying blur. It was a sobering realization that I had done this to myself. That the weakening of my body from fatigue, overexertion, stress, strain and repeated mini back traumas had resulted in this. For years, I had felt soreness in my back and even spent a few Sundays flat out on the couch, but come Monday, I would push through the pain to be the first person back at work. Now, with the hideous shame of an addict, I had to squarely face the lifelong problem I had been ignoring and begin the difficult rehabilitation steps I needed to recover.

Stuck in a hospital bed, I could no longer hide from my addiction to work as I lay motionless, staring at the ceiling. Within days, I was caught up in the vortex of the medical system, filling my body with high doses of drugs and my mind with catastrophic scenarios of a debilitating future. I began a rigorous routine of rehabilitation exercises and physiotherapy. I was hooked up to machines that would send an electric current to my nerves and strapped into traction for hours, adding weights every 30 minutes to spread apart the bones of my spine. They pushed me constantly, trying new things that poked and prodded at my vertebra from every direction. Since I was injured at work, the insidious system was trying to heal me quickly so I could get back on the job. Never once did they just let me rest, slow down or be still.

True to my compulsion to work, I did everything I could to heal as fast as I could. Not just to say I did it, but to prove to everyone that nothing could keep me down. Armed with my new stretching exercises and a prescription for the strongest painkillers available, I returned to work as if nothing had happened, wearing an invisible badge of honor on my sleeve. I ignored any twinges or jolts of pain behind my super pills and marched straight back into the life of a workaholic, cocky and assured of myself. I had beat the odds and I was unstoppable!

The thing about addiction is that the physical symptoms are merely a manifestation of the mental mind. The disproportionate thinking that what you are doing is not hurting you leads to a bigger problem. The justifications and rationalizations in the addict's perceptions of what is healthy and what isn't outweigh the consequences. My mind was convinced I could maintain my pace regardless of the fact that my body was screaming differently. For another decade, I persevered with bouts of debilitating back pain that radiated down into my left leg. For years, I suffered off and on with a limp. I was often unable to drive or even sit due to the contorted posture I needed to assume to avoid the horrific spasms. I needed help getting up out of a chair. Standing up in the morning after hours of laying flat, I suffered excruciating pain. I was unable to lift anything and could not even carry my purse. I walked leaning forward, often losing my balance entirely due to the crippling sensations that would drive a nail of pain into my spine and make my leg cave in. Of course, I kept going, popping my pills and resting just enough to get back to doing whatever task I felt needed doing.

When I became pregnant with my first child, I was bedridden for the last two weeks, unable to lift myself up to eat and needing to stick my butt over the side of the bed to go to the bathroom in a garbage can. Somehow I justified it all, forcing myself to get back up and move despite the physical pain I felt. By the time my second child arrived, I had a full-time nanny to help. I couldn't lift my kids out of their cribs, change their diapers on the floor or breastfeed them in the sitting position. My back had become my Achilles heel, giving out continuously from the stress of building and flipping houses, starting a children's clothing company and managing nine staff working out of my basement. I was a missile pointed straight toward implosion.

Everyone kept warning me of it, but I didn't listen. The discomfort was a constant companion. Pain became normal. I started getting prescriptions for medications that were monitored by the medical system using a triple-page prescription pad and computer tracking system. Once again, I was caught in the coils of my 'acceptable' addiction and the rewarding validation I received from it. Everyone was patting me on the head for my successful life and the *things* that I had. No one knew I had to pee in a cup on the side of my bed because unless my husband helped me, I couldn't go to the washroom in the middle of the night. Only my staff knew I needed them to lift me up from my desk chair at the end of the day. My precious babes cried each time Mommy crumpled to the floor after attempting to pick them up and the nanny was the one to hoist me up off the toilet because I couldn't do it myself.

But hey, I was SUCCESSFUL! I was wealthy, prosperous and acclaimed by many. Except I felt like a weathered scarecrow, stuck on a stick, limbs flapping in the wind with the black crows pecking at my innards, their sharp beaks tearing me apart from the inside out.

The doctors finally told me I needed surgery. They needed to cut into my spine to repair the 20-year-old injury encased in sinew-like scar tissue. It was my only option. The idea of it *terrified* me. I refused. I just continued with my old ways of heat packs, a compression belt and pills as often as was allowed.

Then one day, my daughter stood nervously at my bedside. She knew after years of conditioning not to cause me any pain by accidentally bumping the bed. My nine-year-old son was using all his might to leverage me up so I could drive them both to school. In that moment, I *knew* my problem had reached its pinnacle. My body was giving out on me and I felt terrified of what kind of mother I would be to them in the future. They were both too young to lose me in a risky surgery and had too much life ahead of them to be burdened by my condition.

In that moment, watching my daughter silently worrying and my son trying so hard to help me, I saw my fear mirrored in their eyes. Their palpable concern pushing and straining the very seams of their existence. That night as I lay staring at the ceiling, I knew I couldn't continue living as I was. The years of saying things like, "I can't stand this sore back." and "I'm so sick and tired of this pain." had come true. Those very words, said in anger, *had become my exact reality.* I had perpetuated my problem by repeatedly saying the exact thing I hated. I had become *sick.* I had become *tired.* I *couldn't* stand. Every word was alive in me.

Desperate for a solution, I closed my eyes and prayed to God for another option. I prayed for Him to give me the strength, wisdom and guidance to fix my life without going under the surgeon's knife. That very night, the sound of someone speaking to me awoke me at 4:06 AM, despite my room being dark and empty. The voice said, "Go to Sedona." Sedona? I didn't even know where that was, but the command was so clear and strong that I reached over to the bedside table for my phone and Googled it. Sedona, Arizona was a sacred place for self-healing and nurturing the body-mind connection. It was a land filled with spiritual history and cosmic energy. I stayed up till sunrise reading how world-renowned healers and transformative practitioners flocked to its red rocky vortex to foster and magnify the power of internal energetic healing.

By noon, I had booked myself on a plane. Within a week, I was in a wheel-chair, boarding a plane to immerse myself in a comprehensive retreat centered around healing YOURself. The loving hands that picked me up at the airport and drove me four hours to a healing center — 40 miles off a dirt road and smack dab in the middle of the majestic desert — were the first of many that cared for me during my journey.

At 5 AM the next morning, I was awakened to begin my restorative lifestyle of morning meditation, tapping, Qi Gong, and prayers of gratitude. Pescatarian meals, more prayers and thought re-conditioning were followed by more meditation, time outdoors, and restorative breathing. All were interspersed with chakra activation, yoga, sitting in silence and even more evening meditation. I was taught how to listen. How to hear and reacquaint myself with my body. To connect, discover and meld with every fiber of my Being and every cell of my tissues, muscles and bones. I was shown how I could mentally go inside my body and search out my pain, identify it, label it and lovingly sooth it. I was taught how I could energetically move the molecules of suffering out of my spine and bring in new molecules of vitality. I learned how colors, sound, tempo, vibrations, temperature and recognition gave my pain the opportunity to speak up and share what I had so ignorantly not been willing to hear.

Like a splash of freezing cold water, I felt the jagged shards of anguish about my past shoot to the forefront of my brain. All the stress, hardship and pressure I had burdened my body with flashed like a twisted, fragmented movie in my mind's eye. All the extra work, unattainable expectations and internal demands I had burdened myself with came boiling to the surface like an evil Kraken living under the sea. For the first time, I *saw* my pain. I witnessed the living organism it had become and the vileness it was doing to my structural system, the destruction it was causing *just to be noticed and acknowledged*. It had become an entity within me, with breath and life, frothing to be heard and becoming wickedly debilitating when it wasn't. Up until then, I had always ignored, suppressed and numbed my pain. No one had taught me to embrace it, love it and treat it with care. I had been shown how to mask it, tuck it away or banish it from my thinking. At that healing retreat, I began learning how to listen to what it was trying to tell me. To stop *doing* and instead *be still*. To feel the strength in my breath and the power in my mind to connect with my pain and heal it.

After much prayer and meditation with my forehead on the ground, mentally repairing my body, I was finally able to stand up on my own. I began walking the sacred paths then circling the tiny mystic lake on the property. Soon, I was going on short hikes and making my way to the hilltop for sunrise meditation without the use of the shuttle. I was exercising my mind and body in a symbiotic co-collaboration, listening to it move as if I were a clockmaker fixing its intricate machine by harmonizing the slightest sounds. I became an internal tinker, sitting for hours in silence, meditating, realigning every blood vessel, recalibrating every muscle fiber, fortifying every vertebra, refueling the spinal fluid in every disc, and plumping up the surrounding tissue with a new, healthy life force. I was awakened to the connection I had with both my soul and the container it lived in, recognizing the damage I had wreaked upon it and healing it with the power of my mind.

Much of my work required forgiveness. After 13 difficult years of debilitating back pain, I was finally starting to see the pain for what it was… *a message*. It was the body's way of speaking when the mind stopped hearing the signal. And I needed absolution for my ignorance, restitution for my stupidity. I moved beyond the physical shell and set aside the mental contracts that deemed my workaholism as pleasure instead of pain. I stepped through the portal of preconceived ideas and learned that the value of my skin was not weighted against the results of my efforts. The true essence of my worth emerged. I had gained a deep love for myself and valued my body more than ever.

I returned home, never having to have that invasive surgery. I continued what

I had learned and spent two more years in daily practice, healing my body for hours on end. Today I run, ski, golf, bike ride, horseback ride and even jump on trampolines with my kids — things that were once utterly impossible. I can wrestle with my son and go ice skating with my daughter. I have ziplined in Costa Rica, cliff dived in Spain, skied the Rocky Mountains in Canada and whitewater rafted in Turkey. I have a far richer life than before because I have my health. No physical activity is off limits now. My body is my own and I honor it. I make time to take care of it. I value it as my greatest possession.

In all the years of doctor appointments and rehab clinics, no one ever taught me the body-mind connection or mentioned that I could heal myself. It wasn't until I stepped away from Western medicine and looked at alternatives to restoring my health that I found my way. Now, I am an advocate for those suffering from any ailment to seek out as many OTHER options as you can. Look deeper and search further. Go within and heal not the physical but the emotional. Connect with the problem to find out what the problem is. Forgive yourself from the harm of the past and begin honoring the present, the gift, the beautiful perfection your body is if you just sit silently, and be with it.

Ignite Action Steps

Use affirming words. Words have incredible power. What you say, you create. Too often we say negative things, not paying attention to the harm they cause. Phrases like, "This is killing me." and "That drives me crazy." have a way of materializing when said repeatedly. Try saying, "I'm amazing!" "I've got this!" and "My body knows how to heal itself." Say the things your body needs to hear because it is always listening.

Sit in silence. We can only hear when we decide to listen. Move past the meanderings of the mind and take a trip inside your body. Close your eyes and go within; visit your heart and fill it with love. Bless your stomach, bowels and kidneys. Thank your eyes, ears and nose for working perfectly without you having to command them. See your body as an honored part of you and cherish every inch of it by listening to what it needs.

JB Owen - Canada
Founder of Ignite, World-class Speaker,
International Best-Selling Author and Megapreneur
www.igniteyou.life
 jbowenlovesyou

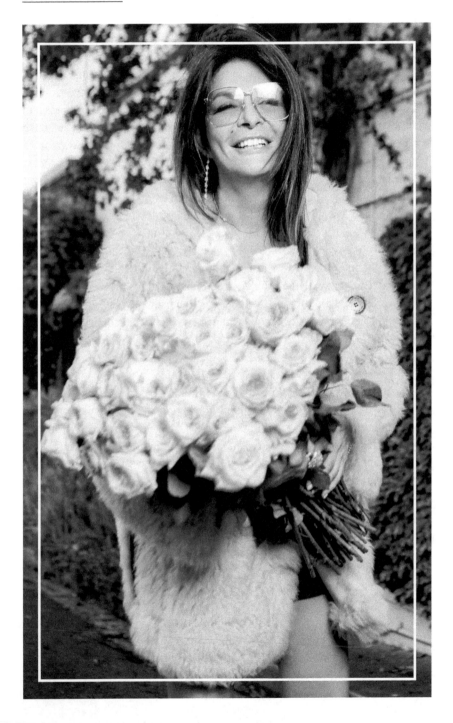

ALEX JARVIS

"Home is where the 'heart' is – put your 'heart' into your home."

My story is about a journey of self-discovery. Realizing that being in harmony with nature and my living space, which I call 'HOME' – played a big part in my Health and Wellness. My intention for you through reading my story is to inspire and encourage you to have fun. Fun by developing a dynamic, flowing continuous space that supports you socially, emotionally, physically and mentally. My desire is to help you develop a sanctuary that reflects who you really truly are.

WHAT A WONDERFUL WORLD

As I looked in the mirror and carefully applied my new *very* red-orange lipstick – a thought popped up in my head – it had been at least a decade ago that I had dared to wear a lipstick that bright in the daytime. 'This was a powerful nightclub red.' The front doorbell rang. I jumped and instantly tightened my belt another notch, around my designer trench coat, putting on my very black, high, patent stiletto shoes.

The show had started – my best friend Claudia stood at my door. Her black Mercedes convertible parked outside. Claudia and I were on a special mission – for the Russian KGB, we both felt the name KGB flowed and sounded better than FSB which is today's name for the Russian intelligence forces – Basia and Sasha being our code names... we were dangerous spies on a TOP SECRET mission. Let the games begin – we were at war. The code word: *Cancer.*

Years before, during our nightclub hopping, we had fun making up our KGB stories entertaining rooms full of potential new boyfriends and becoming very good friends with a Sydney-born Russian called Ollie, who introduced us to the little-known Russian scenes in our corner of Australia: beef stroganoff, Russian dancing, drinking vodka – and an extended community of crazy fun-loving people. Sasha and Basia were always up for silly adventures.

Unexpectedly, I embarked on a new journey and I needed to feel in control of that venture. I knew I had to make up my own 'script' and to act in my very own 'play.' A week before, I had been diagnosed with breast cancer and my head was spinning with all the conversations, choices and solutions given to me by medical staff, friends and family. Everyone seemed to have a story to tell, advice to give and comments to make – but I decided this was my script and that I would be the producer and the director – in its making. Maybe I was in shock or denial (one of the stages of grief) but I actually felt excited, in fact, quite euphoric as I stepped into the moment and embraced fully what was in front of me.

I entered each appointment, medical test or surgery as part of my ultimate mission – which was for the highest good in 'The World of *Basia*.' It was a time that I could stop, be very still and actually give my inner-self, permission to *smell the roses*, be present, and embrace the moment! I began seeing things from a different perspective. Never before had I looked at *self-love and self-awareness* as medicine for recovery.

Looking back into my world six months before my cancer diagnosis – life felt grey and dull – without emotion. I had been so stressed, overworked, overwhelmed and I never stopped. My life felt like it had been shattered into a thousand pieces, by the entrance of a female stalker. During that colorless period, she took great pleasure in tormenting me and smashing all the windows in my home repeatedly. I was living in fear and a nervous wreck (I later found out through police she was a diagnosed Paranoid Schizophrenic). YES, she threatened all my core values and as well my daughter's life and mine. It made sense at the time to board up every accessible window in the house. In the shadows, my fears tripled.

At one point, my daughter and I slept in the car and hotel rooms, until I freed myself from the fear. Finally, I returned to my abode, removed the wooden boards from the windows and let the light back into my house, also letting the joy back into my life. Soon after, I was diagnosed, and my inner journey started with opening up my heart to the light all around me. My home became my palace and sanctuary as I filled it with joy and color. I became aware that to heal the body, I had to first heal my mind. I started to live in harmony in simplistic ways: working with cycles of nature, sleep patterns and food sources from the seasons we were in.

I embraced Aboriginal teachings, believing in the interconnectedness with all life. It felt so connected to my inner knowing, that healing myself required that I restore balance to every area of my life. To be the healthiest me, I started to focus on creating harmony with nature. I found that by creating that space for my health, it elevated me spiritually and by developing that spirituality, it supported my health.

I started seeing things in color and when walking out in nature, I would see the flora and fauna in '3D.' The more I slowed down, decreasing my pace, not forcing anything, just letting things evolve naturally, everything seemed larger than life and more in tune with me. I felt just like the song, my favorite being *I Could Sing a Rainbow* – "Red and yellow and pink and green – purple and orange and blue; I can sing a rainbow. Sing a rainbow, sing a rainbow too."

The beauty of being in the moment and being still gave me the gift of appreciating life for all its wonders, along with a sense of gratitude. I would often say to myself, "Listen with your eyes and listen with your ears..." and then I'd have a feeling of singing from the rooftops. "Sing about everything you see... claiming your voice restores your perceptions of the goodness in this wonderful world."

I engaged in reading all sorts of literature and books, listening to podcasts and watching YouTube. A practice called 'Tzimtzum,' a term used in the Lurianic Kabbalah grabbed my attention. It was the idea of making space for the emergence of something new—*intra*-personally (within ourselves) and *inter*-personally (with others). *Tzimtzum practice means emptying ourselves of ideas, assumptions, judgments as well as any impediments to *being* more... empty. Divine Contraction is defined as 'emptying' in order to make room for the WORLD...

I began to practice this in my own home. My 'KGB days' were now filled with healing from cancer and filling my environment with love. Home to me is any place where you are comfortable and feel as if you can be yourself. A home is a place where you feed off positive energy and feel free. It does not matter whether your home is outside in nature or an apartment in the city, as long as your heart is there. My heart was deep into surrounding myself with the most divine possibilities.

The cancer diagnosis gave me the spirit to fight and create my own story at home and within – the more I took control of my thoughts and responses to things – the more I realized, "We can create our own dream." the more I made it happen.

Over the last nine years, I have had many surgeries. In each hospital room, Andy, my florist, would deliver over a hundred roses every week; the sweet fresh scent of pale pink roses would spread down the corridors of the ward – attracting a continuous stream of visitors from the medical staff. My room was always buzzing with the sound of voices and laughter. The rose-colored pink has the meaning of admiration, elegance, innocence and gratitude. I was truly grateful for giving permission to myself to have what I needed at that time. Those roses were 'me' nurturing 'me,' embracing the ultimate self-care, I allowed myself to be happy and let love in—'self-love.'

I began a second healing path when I fractured three major bones in my ankle and was not able to weight bear for nearly a year. Yes, not being able to walk for *12 months – 365 days*! This meant I slept downstairs and spent 90% of my time confined to my home. Love of color came into play – I surrounded myself with beautiful things, changing the color in the room to suit my mood through rotating artwork, cushions, throws and scarves. It was very uplifting and uplifted me.

I learned the language of color and its magical message made itself known to me. Color has power. It stirred many emotions: stimulated to sedated, excited or calm, feeling hot or cold, irritated or contented, generating feelings of passion and inspiring me spiritually. Color transformed my living environment and increased my productivity, enhanced my social life. Color enhanced my intuition, improving my state of mind and health. My awareness heightened. I felt more alive, excuse the pun, a more colorful human being. Color led me on an unbelievable journey of self-discovery and self-healing.

Words that come to mind when I think of my home now and its design are: creative, fun, whimsical, inventive, dynamic and flowing. I believe that the design of our homes can be used to improve our lives, health and well-being, by using color, sound, and light therapy to enhance the environment. I get great pleasure in coming back to my living space, feeling calm and peaceful. I love the elements of surprise throughout; there are so many new and exciting possibilities each time I walk in my door, contributing to my health and well-being.

I brought the outside in – filled my sanctuary with color and joy. My belief is home is where the heart is – so if it was a hospital room or an overseas trip, living in an AirBNB™, I would have familiar things around me. I would go out to nature, take it all in and bring it back to my home, wearing the energy of the outdoors on my skin. So much joy came from visiting my favorite Moreton

Bay fig tree in a nearby park. It was beautiful and majestic, helping me feel the words in the song by Louis Armstrong, "I see trees of green, red roses too – I see them bloom for me and you…"– color in all forms played such a big part in my healing process.

We all have the ability to create and blossom in a living area that holds a safe space for us to feel loved and secure. The serene color of green is known to bring a feeling of peace and calm. I created my own special piece of green nature in my home in the form of a living wall forming another layer of inter-connectedness around me.

I love the story about the lobster. As it grows, the shell becomes very confining and the lobster finds itself under pressure and uncomfortable. It goes under a rock formation to protect itself from predatory fish, then casts off the shell and produces a new one. Eventually, that shell becomes very uncomfortable so it goes back under the rocks and the lobster repeats the process numerous times. Discomfort is the stimulus that moves the lobster towards growth. However, if the lobsters had doctors, they would never grow, because as soon as it felt uncomfortable, it would go to the doctor for a sedative, then feel fine and never move beyond its shell.

Times of stress are also times of signals for growth and if we use adversity properly, we grow beautifully. Adversity brought me to my biggest Ignite moment – that the answers are within me, and always have been. That I know what I need... and my body shares with me what it needs. I have been on a journey of surrounding myself with pure LOVE and creating the vibration intentionally.

The rose is the highest vibrational flower — the same as love. Most of my adult life, I have looked outwards for my answers. I needed a conduit. The rose essence acts as a 'conscious conduit' to hold space and help navigate the process of looking at my life — letting it unfold naturally. I believe we rise by lifting others, each and every one of us in the community contributes to the ever-evolving journey, engaging, motivating, and inspiring one another, just as the scent of the roses brought hospital staff streaming into my room. With the support of the rose, I felt totally at ease with the experience of continual growth, happening in leaps and bounds. The expansion and connection was so powerful within me and extremely effective as to how I showed up in the community.

The clearer my heart energy was and the more resolved I was with my own story and life issues, the more open I was to positivity, well-being and LOVE in my life. The rose became my guide towards the inner journey to 'create heaven on earth.' KGB missions are now trench coats and red lipstick walking in gardens and smelling flowers. Every week I take a trip to the farmers markets and purchase my scented roses from the growers – changing the color each week from pink, white, deep red, yellow, orange, according to my mood – recently white with a pink center or pale pink has been my choice. It changes the mood within my house. The sweet smell of Rose flower oil every day is diffused throughout my home. And, I think to myself, "What a wonderful world…" Mission accomplished now for 11 years. Yes, I think to myself, "What a wonderful world…" Code word: *Healed*.

I believe we all have our ROSE in one form or another – it could be the strength of your connection with water, plants, gardening, painting, singing, laughing, surfing, meditation, golfing, cooking, cleaning, creating, writing, communicating – these can be support in times of stress. Find your color, fragrance, and joy. Find what means love to you and fill your entire home with it.

Ignite Action Steps

Design and develop a healthier living environment, through a better understanding of the use of color, whatever form works for you. Have you ever wondered why you feel more relaxed when you're in a natural setting? Studies have revealed that the colors in our environment have a direct impact on us. The positive effects of color on mental health relate to the practice of Color Therapy, which uses color as a tool to enhance health. This form of therapy identifies the seven spectrum colors, each having a different type of energy, which corresponds to one of the seven energy centers/chakras of the body. With Color Therapy, for good health and well-being to be achieved, there needs to be a balance between all colors. Understanding color opens our awareness to new dimensions.

There are seven different energy forms in the spectrum of colors.
- *Violet* - is a calming and purifying energy that is believed to also heighten awareness.
- *Indigo* - is identified as having an intuitive energy form that sedates the body and mind.
- *Orange* - is believed to be warming and energizing, as well as stimulating creativity.
- *Blue* - is a calming, healing and relaxing energy.
- *Green* - is attributed to balancing and harmonizing energy. Green is also believed to encourage a deeper understanding and tolerance.

- **Red** - is a stimulating and emotionally exciting energy.
- **Yellow** - is energy that heightens mental activity and alertness, along with promoting confidence.

Shift to the importance of having a good foundation in your life. What's holding you up? What's the container that's solid enough, yet allows you to fly, sway, and where you can experiment with your boundaries and extensions, in a way that has you still feeling rooted and grounded? Your foundation could consist of an exercise routine, family time, filling yourself with inspiration, travel, reading… fill in the blanks for yourself. Create a peaceful foundation free of urgency, where in times of crisis you can go back to foundation… to the roots, where you can slowly expand, and grow.

Questions you can ask yourself. How strong is my foundation? How are my relationships? Do I have rituals, traditions in my life? Do I know who my tribe is? No matter what erupts, the traditions you create will bring you back to your foundation. Practice rituals, traditions and commune with your own tribe. Finding your own routines helps you create a safe space to crawl under your rock and create a larger (shell) container for massive growth in your life and the security to expand experientially.

There are many secrets to a long and happy life. There is much wisdom in the classic saying *'mens sana in corpore sano'* (a sound mind in a sound body). It reminds us that both mind and body are important and that the health of one is connected to that of the other. Give your brain a workout through activities such as crosswords, puzzles, creative pursuits and reading. Seek out activities that appeal to you.

Nurture a long and happy life. Celebrate life each day alone and together with others.

Worry less. Cultivate good habits. Cultivate loving friendships daily. Live an unhurried life. Be optimistic: laugh wherever you go, dance and sing, give thanks every day, keep smiling.

There's no secret to it, really, just LIVE!

Alex Jarivs - Australia
Interior Designer, Rose Alchemist, Speaker, Author, CEO
www.jarvisinteriors.com.au
alex_loveoftherose
jarvisinteriors

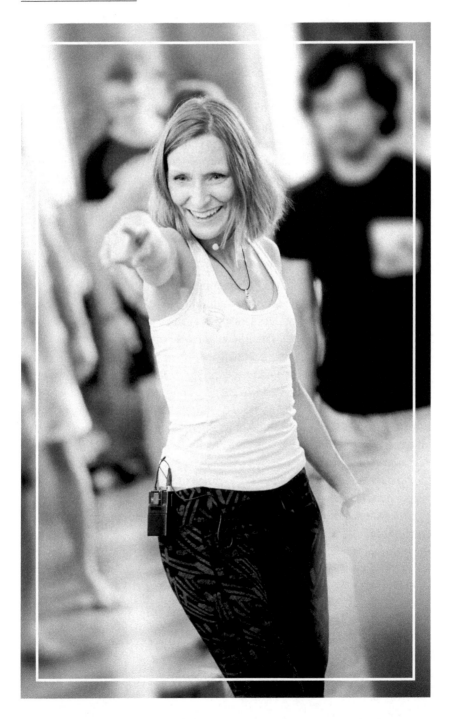

ANNIE LEBRUN

"Move Until Something Shifts."

When it seemed there were no more options around me, I decided to look for answers from the inside. In my search of self-truth and well-being, I bet on life. My wish for you is to tickle your curiosity, to look forward, inward and less outward. To connect with your awareness and to listen to your body. When you find yourself without any solutions, start from within. Your body is made of trillions of cells. It wears you as you wear it. It knows you.

DIVING INTO THE MATRIX - THE INNER WEBBING

If you knew me, you would know that physical freedom is essential for me. I dance, I stretch, I bounce, I jump. Movement is my life: a divine energy flow, an expression of my being. It allows love to radiate from my heart and soul. When sensorily grounded, I feel connected to my mind, to my higher self, to love. To Oneness.

It wasn't always like that. There were two different moments in my life where I felt stuck; these moments built the foundation of who I am today as a person and shifted my vocation. In both cases, I wanted to let go, peel off what was holding me back, those deepest of layers I was wearing. My suits felt like Batman in *The Dark Knight* and then later, *The Wizard of Oz's* squeaky Tin Man. I wanted to release them.

In the first suit, I am sitting on a bench, my eyes fixed on the ants walking on the sidewalk. If the eyes are the mirror of the soul, you would have seen mine knocking on heaven's door, desperately longing to go back to the Source and leave the reality I was trapped in. Even as I took meds to cure the depression, none of the heaviness messing up my head seemed to vanish. During the daytime, it was still night; the pills paralyzed my body in a *Dark Knight* dimension. All I could do was sleep or stare at the walls. On the outside, I was numb; on the inside, it was emotional bursting anarchy. I was angry at the sun for staying up so high, so late. I needed the dark. Mentally stuck, an overwhelming and invasive cloud reminded me that I had no control over my life. I was psychologically misaligned and physically disconnected. I hadn't yet found the inner knowing that would save me.

When it came to my Tin Man suit, I was recovering from an appendix removal. Standing straight or walking longer than 30 minutes took all my energy. I had back and abdominal pain radiating down to my glutes, right knee and ankle, like a disco ball under the flashing strobe light. My gracious mobility seemed to rust a bit more with every week. It kept worsening day by day until, finally, after just 15 minutes of walking, my right leg blocked as if stepping fully into the Tin Man's costume.

After many visits to orthopedic doctors and surgeons, no one could explain my pain and stiffness. They couldn't see it or diagnose it with an MRI, ultrasounds and any other tests. Without an answer to provide, they sent me home and prescribed painkillers, but nothing was killed! The pain and stiffness persisted. I was physically stuck and immobilized completely by the lack of medical options.

In both cases, my suits were crawling under my skin and holding me back: emotionally and physically. In the dark suit, my chest felt heavy; breathing was exhausting with a colossal effort. The Tin Man suit left me staying awake to the shooting disco lights of pain and made every step into the living a bit more difficult. The physical challenges affected the psychological and the other way around too. In both situations, I ended up receiving more drug prescriptions, and just like a hot potato, each time I was sent back home, clueless. F**k!

Even at the lowest points on that park bench watching ants, accepting NO or CAN'T as an answer was NEVER a part of my agenda. Yes, I am a rebellious type! Even back then, I wanted to improve my health issues, my anxiety and my lack of movement. I wanted to release the pain and the restrictions from both Batman and the Tin Man.

I wanted to MOVE ON and GET UNSTUCK. In my emotional state, it was hard to describe what was going on with me. Words were meaningless to explain that overwhelmingly heavy weight. There must be a way? Or a key? I wanted to break those patterns... habits... or whatever it was that I was caught in! My gut feeling was whispering to me, "No!" In fact, it was screaming.

Each time, my body reminded me that it had the last word. Fine, I agreed to listen. I couldn't avoid it anymore, the noise became too loud, the strobe lights of the disco ball assaulted me and I had to surrender. I could no longer ignore the whispers that became screams. If emotional states communicated with biological responses, they were mirroring what was going on deep inside. If the problems were felt from within, the solution would be there too. I dove into my matrix. I had to listen, to observe, to contain, especially when I thought I was losing my mind. My physical and emotional reactions were messing with my head.

Maybe there was a purpose to all this? Maybe thinking less and feeling more would be the answer? I had nothing to lose up to that point. If our skin works like our kidneys, I reasoned, and all those feelings and constraints were crawling under my skin, I was going to sweat the depression and the shitty medications right out of me.

So, I started to move. I did weights; I did kickboxing. I knocked open the box and stepped out, starting to shift my senses outside the dark suit. That inner knowing that I was alive, yet did not feel alive, triggered my stubbornness. I knew I had to get out from under that dark cloud and face the light again. I couldn't continue that way. Have I tried everything possible? Was there another option left? Somehow, the movement... called me home to myself. *That was the key.* The physical numbness faded. Finally, I could feel... my body reset... senses alive again... calming the emotional flows with dopamine.

Stepping out of that dark fog, refusing the medications, I trained fanatically five to six times a week. Sweat was weakness rising out of me, leaching out the chemicals. I started to connect with my senses and felt gradually stronger and bolder. My head raised over my shoulders; my vision of life slowly shifted!

I observed the green of tree leaves, tasted my food differently, went to pet shops caressing and interacting with animals. Touch became my new language. I listened to the world with my hands. They would interpret life differently. I could know people, feel them, listen to them, connect with them through touch. I was tapping into a new world as well as my own. I realized my senses were working through my hands, detecting and perceiving what my eyes and my ears would miss. I was on the move, thirsty for more awareness and deeper connections, opening my heart for new meanings in life, connecting with my Matrix. Yes, it was making sense! The Batman suit had vanished.

I began learning about anatomy and physiology; I discovered a new approach to viewing the human body: the connective tissue. For centuries, biologists, physicians, doctors and surgeons didn't pay much attention to this system. They thought this white stuff's purpose was just to wrap muscles and bones. While considered unsexy and no superheroes, pathologists systematically got rid of the 'scrap' while dissecting cadavers. Without giving much attention, they threw the waste away, confusing the white swan with the ugly duckling.

Fascia, or connective tissue, is the biological fabric holding you together. It's made of collagen and elastin proteins existing within a gel fluid called the *ground substance*. The fascia is everywhere, wrapping every individual cell into a bag, grouping cells into another bag, forming muscles, joints and organs. It organizes our inner suit into layers from the bones reaching all the way up to under our skin. I like to compare our inner body to the Russian matryoshka stacking dolls of many layers. You can also look at a slice of grapefruit to see how everything is held as one within the tiny segments.

It is just recently that the international medical fields have joined forces and decided to give a little bit more attention to the white swan. The First International Fascia Research Congress happened in 2007. Physicians, bodyworkers, physiotherapists, researchers, biologists and orthopedists met in Boston. The ugly duckling had become a superhero!

Meanwhile, living in Germany and being so close to all the new fascia research and development, I was able to attend courses about a new concept, *Faszientraining*. I learned how the biological fabric could be trained physically. Wow! Could I reshape my inside and turn back time? I rapidly integrated the training concepts and theory into my manual therapy. The beauty of it brought me hope. I could improve and care for my connective inner webbing! Mobility was my new youth.

As I learned about this new medical system, my perception of the body changed completely. The multitasking fascial tissues are the web of tension and compression suspending the bones. The fascia wears many suits: the connector, the stabilizer, the protector, the movement facilitator, the organizer and the communicator. It is highly sensitive and communicative. The vast majority of our sensory neurons are located in the 'skin of everything.' The fascia has a sense of its own; it is your physical map, your body's internal GPS that connects the brain to your body.

I began to realize that we are not constructed like buildings. Motion comes from a floating compression, not the bones. Just as Galileo had to convince the people of his time that the earth was round, not flat, we need to see that bones are part of our liquid system. We are really just a system of cells holding all the tissue together. Fascia organizes our insides to keep our toe cells with our feet and our heart cells in our chest. In your mother's womb, this tissue shaped you before you had organs or even a heart.

My *Faszientraining* oiled my Tin Man suit. I trained and self-treated with foam rollers and many myofascial release tools. I realized that my body's restrictions came from scar tissue due to my post-surgery side effects. But I also had other stiffness coming from old repetitive postural patterns.

While working patiently on the adhesions around my abdominal scars and breaking the pattern from my compensatory postures, I released the radiating pain along my leg and reduced my lower back tension. Agility and ease returned to my walk. The more I brought attention to my body, the more I shifted into fluid and gracious movements.

While on the quest to search for my inner truth, I realized that the inner biological design was my new buddy and it had a super talent: to bounce! As kids, we used to jump around so easily and non-stop. Our whole internal fascial structure was flawless. Over time, due to poor posture, scoliosis, trauma, lack of flexibility, repetitive strain, chronic inflammation and surgical scars, our fascia becomes tight and restrictive; it thickens. Day after day, week after week, we ingrain patterns and postural habits and mold our bodies. As a result of the postural misalignments, tension squeezes out the watery, jelly-like system, causing body parts to dry out. We shrink in three dimensions. And that is the new definition of aging! I had a new life motivation: staying young!

With eccentric, dynamic stretches, adding bounces, I could train my fascial elasticity! I was now *bouncing back*! As I experienced myofascial bodywork and training, I noticed how awareness was the key to my physical and mental wellbeing. The more I focused on body sensations while training, stretching and moving, the more I connected to myself. I observed my body restrictions. It felt like a spotlight highlighting my body parts; my brain would interact with them and resocialize. It seemed I could feel them reviving, at first with pain, just like frozen fingers warming up, coming back to life. Through refined movements guided with my awareness and my breathing, I concentrated on the painful first encounter and listened. The pain would dissipate, leaving space for the flow, a warm breeze, feeling relief and lightness. As my layers were sheering and gliding with new hydration, Tin Man defrosted further. I was tapping into my protective physical and mental shield, calibrating the parasympathetic and sympathetic nervous systems.

Becoming bolder influenced not only my posture but my behavior too. Postures transmute behaviors. Over the years, we physically shrink and, coincidentally, lock unconscious beliefs, reflexes and patterns in the deep tissue layers of our inner suit. You become how you stand, sit and do. Making our-selves posturally small (stress, lack of movement, sitting down) creates physical misalignments and tensions, and shapes our fascial network.

As a result of living with constant stress and the production of stress hor-mones, we continue to function just in survival mode despite the first signs of discomfort. We grow accustomed to the pain as the brain just wants us to function and, in that mode, we adopt postural and physical behaviors molded inside. The body talks to us every second, but we are so into our heads, routines and the modern-day stress, like being trapped inside the Wizard's tornado, we move away from our senses. Our body needs to talk louder and louder until the pain becomes non-negotiable, insisting on our attention. First signals sent — tensions, soreness, tightness. Not listening? The next warning will ramp up — raising the stakes with increased pain, vertigo and additional lack of mobility. But the pain is not an overdue notice or a death sentence. It is a signal! Your body is begging for attention, for connection, for awareness. Hey buddy—*move*!

Ignoring all the signs creates a distortion of who we are, and with time, our brain will pick up and accept the repetitive postures or gestures. It wires the data after 100,000 times. It will eventually feel normal. The good news is that, the more I created the movement that suited me, and repeated that new *me*, the more my brain adopted this healthy way of being.

I hope this glimpse into my 'inter-connected' journey has shown you how important overall mental and physical wellness is. I hope you are inspired to be more you, more connected, more in the present moment. How about showing your bolder side, the real you? The inner you. Your mind and body can become one. Inner connectedness is your boldness. Oneness is living! Dive into it!

IGNITE ACTION STEPS

- **Dust off your foam roller.** Release your trigger points, your tensions. Foam rolling helps to reestablish proper movement and reduces pain in restricted body areas. No pain, no gain? Yes, a bit true, but it's one of the best ways to unravel and unwind your inner design and free your motion.

- **Feeling is knowing:** Our brain will always want to avoid pain. When we start to unravel our biomechanical distortions, pain is perceived very differently from one person to another. There are benefits to feeling pain if we align ourselves earlier, observe and make changes. Thomas W. Myers mentioned, "Pain is a condition, the motor intention to withdraw accompanying the sensation." If you are not running from it, it is just a sensation. To be able to release, you have to be willing to feel. The pain and sensations are your guidelines telling you: you are freeing nerve endings but also releasing biomechanical and emotional patterns and paths. Dissociating emotions from physical feelings helps you to observe and let go.

- **Biochemistry:** Change your biochemistry within minutes. Try 'power posing'— striking a Superhero's posture of confidence. Within 120 seconds, your testosterone goes up 20 percent and decreases cortisol 15 percent.

- **Head to toe:** For lower back pain or headaches, roll your feet on tennis balls for two to five minutes to stimulate your whole fascia. For chronic pain or seasonal mood swings, roll three to five minutes every day for three weeks to positively decrease pain and stabilize mood.

- **Break the habit** of the monkey-turtle chair posture! Very challenging in our modern times! Sit on your sit bones, the edgy part of your hips. Notice how your belly button is slightly pulling in on its own. Show a little bit more of your heart; it balances your head back to its original place. Keep this pose as long as you can. If this feels weird, good!

- **Rewire your brain with your eyes.** Instead of staring at your phone while walking, unaware, look straight ahead. Why? Try this. Stand up, feet hips wide apart, look down for ten seconds. Then, fix a point straight ahead of you as if you were driving. Is your weight shifting back on your heels, grounding you to your pelvis and feet? Be bold and boost your posture within a blink of an eye.

- **Joy is an expandable motion.** Just play your best music in your headphones and dance. Joy always shakes your whole being. Expand yourself. Go tiger!

Annie Lebrun - Germany
Founder, Body-Matrix Specialist
www.bodymatrixspecialist.com
bodymatrixspecialist
BODYMATRIXSPECIALIST

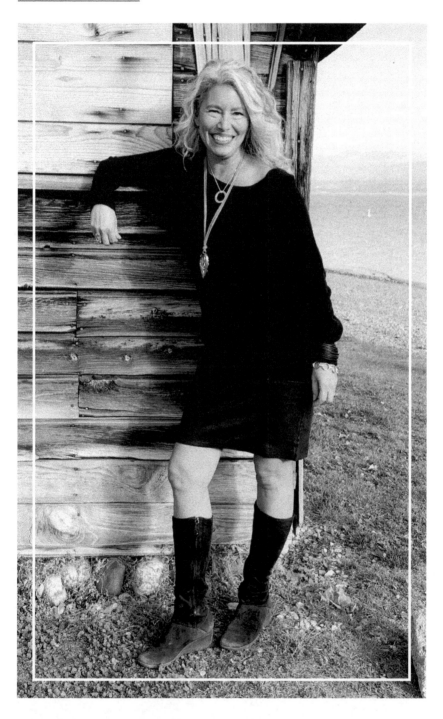

Shannon Bliss

*"A love that we have felt so deeply, we can never lose;
it becomes part of us."*

**It is my hope that by reading my story you start to see beyond your grief.
Remember you are not alone. Let the memories of your loved ones inspire
you to carry on and make a positive impact on those around you.**

BLISSED Love

It's been nine months since Alan left. I first spotted him while I was waiting
to board my flight from Carlsbad to Los Angeles. I was getting my son Shaydon
settled in Carlsbad, California after his recent injury. Alan seemed to be in a
heated discussion with a fellow I'd seen staggering out of an open air bar just
minutes before. Overhearing a bit of their conversation, I surmised the intoxicated fellow was from England. My late husband Tony was from England so
it was an easy accent for my ears to decipher.

I remember being annoyed. I really didn't want to leave my son in Carlsbad, but I had clients back home who needed me too. After what felt like an
exhausting wait, I boarded. While getting settled, that same intoxicated fellow
became verbally abusive to our beautiful African American flight attendant
who strongly stood her ground. The plane was halted not once but twice — it
was only two years after the tragedy of 9/11 and poor behavior by anyone was
not tolerated. My connection was tight and with those delays, I knew I had
missed my next flight. Upon landing, I headed straight for the United Airlines

counter. Alan, who only a few minutes earlier, had sprinted from the plane, was in line in front of me, speaking animatedly in his incomprehensible Scottish brogue to a tiny clerk who I could see struggling to understand him. Listening, I heard his destination was the same as mine. Still annoyed and wanting to get my flight resolved, I stepped in and saved the day. This was the beginning of a new chapter of my life.

But I'm getting ahead of myself. Let me take you back to where my journey began.

It was the spring of 2007. Tony, Shaydon and I were on a zipline adventure in the little tourist town of Jaco, Costa Rica. We were a week into our vacation and I was starting to get accustomed to the humidity, but Tony still seemed to be struggling. I had been concerned about Tony even before we left on holiday as he seemed off... forgetful... which troubled me as he was a stickler for details. Once we began our aerial descent through the rainforest, the surreal beauty captured me and my worries were forgotten, at least for the time being.

We rented an SUV so we could go exploring for the second half of our trip. Tony seemed tired and thought it best I drive... odd... another alarm bell was going off in the back of my mind. Tony loved to drive and I'd rather not, but driving through the hills was a thrill and driving a standard kept my mind focused on the task at hand.

After two weeks of the beauty and majesty of the rainforest, we arrived back home to the urban city of Oakville, Ontario where we'd lived for the past six years. We resumed our busy lives; life was full and we were happy.

The very next Saturday marked the start of Shay's bowling league season and it was our family ritual outing, although Tony seemed to have the flu, so we left him in bed to rest. Shaydon was a natural bowler and was having a great game. Part way through, I saw Tony arrive, but something was wrong. His gait was off and his left arm looked heavy. I went to meet him and have a better look, trying to remain calm. Up close, I saw the left side of his face was drooping and he had limited control of his arm. I had to get him to Emergency.

I knew this was going to be a battle as he wasn't a fan of hospitals. Born in Cheltenham, England in 1952, he was one of the last children to contract polio. He underwent numerous surgeries and was left with a limp. Luckily, he had a strong-willed mother who taught him that he could overcome any obstacle. Like his mother, Tony was a strong and determined presence. He could light up the room with his smile and everyone loved him, especially me.

Against Tony's will, I got him into the car and we went to Emergency. Somewhere, I found time to call a friend who was a radiology nurse at the local hospital and explained the situation. She had a team waiting for us when we arrived. A whirlwind of tests later sent us hastily to another hospital for an emergency MRI. Life as we knew it was about to change forever.

We sat in the hospital room waiting for the results, not fathoming what our futures held. A small man with dark curly hair introduced himself as Tony's neurosurgeon, here to speak to us about his results. The conversation that followed is vague in my memory. I remember feeling a surge of electricity go through my body and then feeling numb with fear. I heard the doctor say, "An aggressive brain tumor that needs to be removed immediately. Are all of Tony's affairs in order?" We were both in shock.

Everything felt rushed. The surgeon wanted to do an awake craniotomy surgery on Monday at the latest.

During the surgery, I sat in the waiting room and my thoughts took me back to how we met. I remember when I first locked eyes with Tony. It was 1989 and I had applied for a job at the local truck dealership. It was interview day and I was nervous. I felt someone smiling at me as I walked through the front doors, when I looked over, *there he was*. This handsome man with well groomed chestnut hair, locks of curls that slightly hung over his collar, was standing behind a large office window. His smile calmed me... it was love at first sight. A few years passed before we came together as he was from Corporate and it was taboo to date, but love always finds a way.

Yet here I was sitting in a hospital waiting room, wondering what was going to come next. Despite all our worry, Tony came through it with his usual spark and jest. He was the ideal patient and all the nurses loved him.

Recovery was surprisingly much quicker than I imagined. We resumed our lives within a few short months. From the beginning, Tony's prognosis was not great and I had so many questions for his doctors with very few answers. The lack of knowledge haunted me... how did they not know how this all started? Was there nothing we could do to prolong his life? Therapies? Nutrition? Anything? All my thoughts and suggestions were shot down, but I was determined to find help.

My research landed on Holistic Nutrition. This is where I found HOPE. I knew I had to take charge, so I signed up for classes. I was 41 and terrified. Could I actually do this? Would I pass? Could I make a difference? How was I going to manage work, studies, my family, Tony's health, and still find time for the things I loved? Was I nuts? I have no idea how I pulled it all off, but with flying colors, I did.

Two years passed. We both were under the illusion that he was in the clear, but one fateful day, an MRI showed another tumor. It was time to pack up and head home to our family for what looked like our final days. By Christmas, Tony's decline was very noticeable. Increasing tiredness, slurred speech, difficulty walking... in early spring, Tony had two more surgeries. It was a difficult time but we got through it as the family banding together.

Tony passed May 19, 2010. I will always remember his wit, radiant smile, the kindnesses he exuded to others, and his spark. The interesting mismatched attire he chose to wear on the weekends that made me laugh... and most of all the love that made me feel I was enveloped in a protective bubble.

After losing Tony, putting one foot in front of the other seemed a chore. When I thought of the person he was... a great man, always giving, always so brave, always challenging us to be better people... he inspired me throughout our lives together and the memory of him inspired me to carry on.

There's something about Saturdays. It was a Saturday morning a few years later and my home phone was ringing... the answering machine clicked on and I heard a womans' voice, something about a hospital, could I call her back!?! I quickly listened to the message again. My son had been in an accident at work. In shock, I called the number and the nurse who had left the message answered the phone.

Shaydon was working as a welder with a company that was retrofitting a sawmill in Radium Hot Springs. He had fallen 18 feet onto his back and was being airlifted to hospital. The nurse asked me if I would like to speak to him. My heart was racing when she put him on the phone. I could hear the fear and pain in his voice. He was getting increasingly upset, saying he couldn't feel his legs.

I mustered all the strength I had to help calm him, reassuring him he was going to be okay. He was in good hands and I'd be there as fast as humanly possible. The nurse spoke to me again, explaining they couldn't give him anything for pain yet. During the flight to the trauma center, he had gone into arrhythmia and a defibrillator was needed to normalize his heartbeat... WHAT? He was only 24! I wanted to scream and cry at the same time, but that wasn't going to help.

I arrived at the hospital a few minutes after my cousin Maryanne. She had just driven five hours from the opposite direction to be there for us. No sooner had we arrived at the hospital than Shaydon's surgeon spoke with us. Shaydon was in bad shape. Both eyes were bruised and swollen; a neck brace and some sort of traction was needed for back support. It was a spinal cord injury. It took everything for me to hold it together. He had to be okay; we were inseparable.

I wouldn't let myself think anything negative as he was wheeled into surgery.

We were in the waiting room when Tony's daughter Sarah arrived. We seemed to be old hands at this torturous waiting game. The love and support of family in difficult times makes all the difference in helping us to survive these ordeals and hold on to hope.

It was a long journey of rehabilitation. Shaydon worked hard at recovery, enrolling in a spinal cord boot camp in Carlsbad. The moment Shay entered the bright airy gym, his wheelchair was put off to the side and the process of learning how to work out as a parapalegic began. The gym atmosphere was positive and encouraging. People of all ages from all over the world were seeking help and moving forward. It was a place of HOPE for not just Shaydon, but for myself as well.

After helping him settle, it was time to say our brave goodbyes as I headed to the airport and home. I had been trying to control my mood all morning, trying to hide my tears. I didn't want to leave my only child in this strange place. What if something happened or he needed me, and I was thousands of miles away? But thinking like this wasn't going to give him the courage to get through this. Tough love and the memory of Tony's strength had gotten us this far.

I arrived at the airport only to be told there was a delay. This just added more fuel to my sad and sour mood. I could have spent more time with Shaydon! It wasn't long before other passengers started to fill up the waiting room. Still annoyed at life, I picked up my phone so I could avoid eye contact. A heated conversation broke my thoughts and I looked up… and this takes me back to the beginning of my story. The English fellow I had seen staggering out of the bar and this other man with the thick Scottish accent and long blonde hair any woman would be envious of… Alan.

After rescuing him at the United Airlines counter, we had a couple hours in LAX to kill. It had been an emotional day thus far, so Alan offered to buy me a glass of wine. He was full of colorful stories of his past in Scotland and was in the process of setting up a business in Carlsbad. He was so easy to be around, like we'd known each other for years, and I knew from the moment we spoke there could be something between us.

Even so, I wasn't emotionally ready for that. A friend maybe… but I needed to stay focused for Shay and his recovery.

Alan and I met for coffee once or twice before I was to head back to California. Project Walk, Shay's spinal cord boot camp, was having a televised function I was meant to attend that afternoon. Knowing my plans, Alan booked to fly the day after me. But then my phone rang at 4 AM. My flight was cancelled due to fog that was expected to last days. I was so disappointed. Alan messaged me early that morning to wish me a safe journey. I explained the situation and he wasted no time cancelling his flight. We drove together to California that afternoon, my knight in a shiny white XJ8 Jag. We talked the entire journey, getting to know each other's thoughts, experiences and values. That was the beginning of Alan and I.

Our lives were full with family, friends, music, parties, visits to Scotland, and so much love until one day he had a pain in his lower abdomen. He first felt it doing leg ups during a workout and thought he had pulled a muscle. It wasn't long after that he was diagnosed with bowel cancer with no option for surgery.

That sinking feeling I had felt with Tony and then Shaydon hit me once again.

Chemotherapy started. His first few treatments seemed to do him wonders, then the side effects started. Nausea, lack of appetite, weight loss, but what seemed to trouble him the most was the loss of his long blonde hair.

Alan was determined to beat the disease; he didn't want to leave his family and so wanted to see his granddaughters grow up. So he put on a brave face and persevered.

January 6th was check up day with his oncologist. His latest blood work and MRI reports were encouraging. We headed home with HOPE, only there was still pain at a drain site for the ascites. Three days later, he didn't have the energy to leave his bed.

Alan passed not a month later, surrounded with the love of his family and friends.

I have been 'BLISSED,' like my last name, with true love not once, but twice and with the unconditional love of a child. I could easily sit and wallow in pain, or I could make a conscious choice to celebrate the beautiful memories of the inspiring men in my life. I choose to celebrate BLISS.

Life is a cycle that many people do not want to face. We all have a purpose here. Mine is a life of service. As a Nutritional Practitioner, I often see people stuck in GRIEF. The memories of how I survived my grief comes to mind. Accepting help from my friends and family was huge. I let them care for me. I let them cook and do the mundane chores of everyday life so I could be free to heal. Even though I'm fiercely independent, I have learned that my health and wellness depends on letting people help me.

As you grieve, remember your family and friends are also grieving. Let them in. Try to resume your regular life as soon as you have energy. You can start slowly and, as the days pass, you can accomplish more. Sleep is impera-tive for a positive day, so make sure you're getting enough. Eat healthy, drink plenty of water, and find reasons to build joy even in grief, even if only for a moment. Talk about your loss when you feel strong enough to let GRIEF trickle in. You will have good days and bad days, so expect that. Let your memories INSPIRE you to go forward. Remember you're not alone. Asking for help is a sign of strength, not weakness.

In loving memory of the great men I've had in my life, Anthony Paul Bliss, my husband, and Alan William Stirling, my partner, they will forever be missed. May the thoughts of them keep inspiring friends and family to be their very best, do right by others and share an infectious smile to brighten others' lives.

IGNITE ACTION STEPS

- Accept help from friends and family. Remember they, too, are grieving. Helping you helps them through their grieving.

- Rest, everything is better after a good sleep. It is imperative for a positive day.

- Talk about your loss to friends, family or a counselor.

- Nourish your body with healthy food. Drink plenty of water and limit stimulants like caffeine and alcohol.

- Exercise and create some happy endorphins.

Shannon Bliss - Canada
Certified Nutritional Practitioner
www.healthisbliss.ca

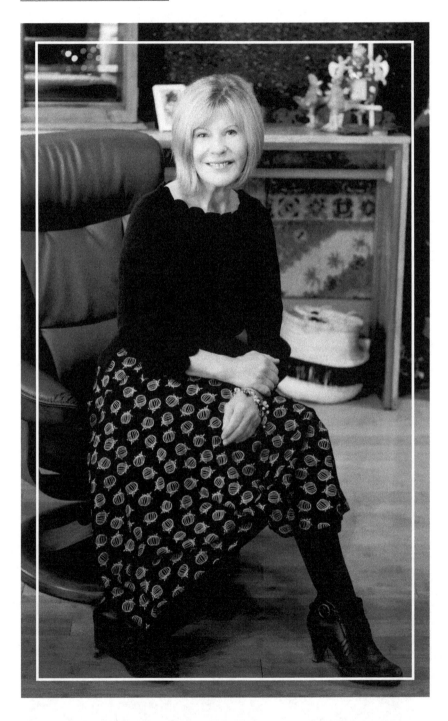

DIANNA DELACOEUR

"When you feel as if life has let you down, either through laughter or tears, give your heart fully and trust that the real gifts will be uncovered."

In sharing this story of my daughter, whose disabilities at birth became the fulcrum for change in my own life, it is my wish to inspire others in finding strength and hope to overcome the difficult challenges life sometimes surprises us with. Remember that life is often mysterious; what we might initially perceive as a negative event, once unfolded, hides gifts that reveal a deeper message.

LIFE'S TRICKS AND TREATS

There in the maternity ward at the small hospital, cheerful Halloween decorations were posted all throughout. Pumpkins, friendly ghosts and little black cats adorned the walls. I wondered, alone in the night, if this was a trick or treat presented for me and my baby, born on the cusp of Halloween? My life had suddenly shattered like billions of shimmering shards of glass. Grief and pain overwhelmed me. Was this some sort of nightmare I would wake from? Was this a sick joke? Was the Universe laughing, I wondered? Why me? Why my baby? I had joined a gym, took daily walks, vitamins and supplements. I had done all the 'right things' that I could think of. I, who had so looked forward to my surprise child.

Hot water beat relentlessly down on me, like tiny, sharp knives fiercely blasting my face. I sobbed; I shouted and banged my head against the spotlessly white, glistening walls in a moment of privacy where I didn't have to pretend. My whole world had abruptly shifted in direction, slamming on the brakes and putting an end to my dreams, and I cried, "What are you doing God?" I crumpled, dropping to my knees there in the shower, welcoming physical pain to ease my inner agony. "Why MY baby?"

It felt like a scythe cutting through, cleanly ending any magic in my life. A crumbling marriage was one thing, but this, tonight was the culmination, a true kick in the teeth. I was insulated, now, from the necessity for polite smiles. They were no longer required as they had been back in that hospital room shared with another mother. A happy mother. A mother who beamed and could cradle her newborn, tucked safely in her arms.

My baby, my little girl who had entered the world with hydrocephalus and spina bifida, had immediately been whisked away from me down long, unfamiliar halls and behind impersonal, cold metal doors. After her birth, I had been given only minutes to breathe in the velvety sweetness of her skin, to look with awe into those deep blue eyes. Instead of my daughter, I was given only papers and more papers to sign, releasing her to be transferred, so tiny and vulnerable, to an ambulance which carried her even further away from me to another hospital. There would be no mother allowed to ride with her, to touch or comfort her, no father, not even a grandmother or friend. There was no one for her but me, and here I stayed — cloistered in that shower, my only private space to cry out my frustration and impatience. It was taking too long for my own discharge papers to be completed so that I could follow her.

My mind would not quiet. "Why me?" Had there been something in the water? Could it have been the poisons, sprayed to halt the weeds by the road-sides? Had I unknowingly been exposed to some teratogenic chemical? I tried so hard! I had been so careful! Why did this happen to my baby? My beautiful baby, an innocent child! What kind of a God are you?! I cursed, pressed against that unyielding wall. I felt my whole life dissolving, slipping, sliding away in fear, anger and despair.

Finally, somehow, a calmness, a sense of understanding and acceptance seemed to mercifully and gently envelope me, illuminating and abating the wild thoughts of my crazy mind. I remembered a dream I had had some months ago in early pregnancy. In this dream, I looked down to see my womb like crystal, trans-parent, slowly revolving. Inside lay my baby, floating in the amniotic waters… but there had been something wrong with her legs. That had been very clear.

Not long after that dream, I had stopped idly in front of a bookstore window one morning, one hand on my pregnant belly. The book *Everything That Could*

Go Wrong With Your Baby was on display. I wondered who would even write such a book. So negative! I knew no one who had a disabled child. Still, I bought the book and read it. And when my daughter was born, I knew immediately upon seeing the angry red blister on her spine what had transpired.

Standing there in the shower, the memory of that dream arose and time seemed to soften, then to stop for me. How could I have forgotten about that dream? I realized in that moment I was not alone, and I had not *been* alone. Like breath in air suspended, the energy shifted.

In the stillness of my anguish, the pain faded and I no longer felt alone. That dream and that book had been a gift which helped prepare me for this new life. A hush of peacefulness surrounded me, like all encompassing wings holding me, no more words or thoughts. My questions had drifted away, revealing inner quiet in my heart. A mystery which needed no more cerebral understandings.

Surrender, like a cloak, silenced the frantic thoughts of my mind. In the solitude of that small shower, somehow determination blossomed and grew. I could not continue feeling sorry for myself. Why was I really crying? Because I had no power to heal her? I would never be able to take her load and carry it myself. Who was I to feel so cheated? Whose was the real burden? Hardly my own.

Her needs and joy were paramount; my role was to support her in her growth, healing and living as 'normal' a life as possible. For me, this was a reminder that healings come in many forms: perception and choice, positive or negative. You can become a victim of circumstances or choose to take another path.

A myriad of words filled my mind and I put them to paper.

A Question of 'Perfection'
The first time I saw you daughter,
You lay there, eyes opening,
blue laser beams slicing through my heart.
I knew in that instant I would never be the same.

Like a rose opening on film, in slow motion
Petals unfurling, reaching for the sun...
But touched by an early frost...
Forever frozen, unable to spring free.

They told me daughter (being young yet)
I could always try again...
Might even achieve perfection on a second round

But I ask you - I ask you
What is the meaning of 'perfection'
And does it lie in the eye or live in the heart?

Hearing my words, they were struck dumb
Sterile and white, they turned their backs and fled.

I wondered your thoughts on this, as my finger traced the curve of your ear.
Delicate as a seashell nestled in the waves of your hair.

O daughter, you are my flower

And if petals seem sometimes less than perfect
Who can tell me what is "perfect"?
I am here to say
You are perfect to me.

What I had not known on that day was that, though my life and dreams had been forever changed, though my heart and mind ached, I was being presented with so many hidden gifts. Our lives would be forever moving forward. If we fell, we would get up and keep going because there was no turning back.

Becoming pregnant at 20 had been a promise of new beginnings. I dreamt of a storybook life for my child. I imagined all of the things we could do together.

Those first few hours after my daughter's birth seemed like an impossible illusion.

Once my mind had calmed, I realized I was a mother to a new human being who was completely dependent on me for her life and her future. Something new came alive within me. Spurred forward and ignited into action, in spite of the lack of a background in formal education, I fearlessly enrolled in college with my goal set on the medical field, either in nursing or becoming a physician. I was determined to learn and provide compassionate medical care for my daughter and other children and families. I was resolved to teach, support and demand respect for those who needed help.

I started out in a local college then transferred out of state to the University of Washington for pre-med studies. Throughout the days and evenings, I rushed from class to class across campuses. I worked weekends and nights struggling to make ends meet, falling asleep to taped lectures and juggling caring for a baby whose shunt constantly malfunctioned, who was stricken with meningitis and needed repeated hospitalizations. My stress levels rose.

When an acceptance into one of the nursing programs I had applied to arrived in my mailbox, I stopped to catch my breath. Should I continue on towards a medical degree or enter the nursing program? I wanted to give my all, but who was I giving my all to? After some deep soul searching I made the decision to move back to California to attend nursing school.

My daughter's needs and her countless surgeries forced me to redefine my life and reset my goals. Her presence compelled me to reevaluate everything I had ever learned about religion, spirituality and God. Because of her, I found a new vision of God, one of compassion and wisdom. I discovered a God who does not 'punish' or 'reward.' A God who asks of us to give our all and play this game of life through to the end with everything we have. With open hearts, sometimes on bloody knees when we have no idea how to rise again yet find ourselves standing. A God who teaches in ways that often seem incomprehensible through what I have come to call The Great School of Life, a school that never ceases until the breath stops.

Inspired by my daughter, I began studying different religions and Eastern philosophies. We traveled together to India several times, meeting both famous and less renowned spiritual teachers. We visited various ashrams, missions and sacred spots. She made friends with everyone she met, while I studied different healing modalities. On our return to the United States, this continued.

I undertook studies and training in Hatha and Raja yoga. Later, my daughter stayed with her best friend and cousin in Seattle while I studied at the Theosophical Society on Orcas Island. A few years after, I was initiated as a Reiki Master, then continued on to create a conglomeration of alternative healing techniques of my own. During these bright years, my daughter often accompanied me and was herself initiated into Reiki and various modalities of energy healing. Without her, so many experiences and awakenings would have passed me by, unaware. Those were years that granted us a time of magic and grace, through struggles, laughter and tears.

That long ago Halloween night, I had thought my life was falling apart. That day, my version and vision of 'perfection' changed. I was blind to the hidden gifts awaiting — so many awesome gifts were given to me. This daughter who, in spite of multiple and ongoing warnings to the fragility of her life, even to her imminent demise — continued on. She lived, in spite of the weeks of coma with meningitis as a toddler, in spite of years of multiple repeated surgeries for shunt failures, even in spite of the onset of seizures as she entered puberty.

She walked everywhere she pleased like a drunken sailor with her rolling gait, heedless of the future of wheelchair dependence promised by authorities. She relented to leg braces and, on the rare occasion, to crutches. She kept to her own path with determination, her chin up, ignoring humiliations, refusing to give them power over her.

Her life was rich and full. She attended church dances in high school, rode horses, loved the 'wild concerts' of India's holy woman, Amritanandamayi Ma, and often sat rubbing her feet during darshans. She insisted on rebelling as a teenager, as all teenagers do. She eloped with a man 20 years older than she was and had babies 'just like everyone else.' She experimented in life, learning through her own choices, defying the odds for years into adulthood. She drove me totally bonkers at times with worry, but she insisted on living as fully as possible in her own independent way.

Her death was constantly predicted throughout her life, but in the end, it was finally due to a hit and run driver, not her disabilities. It took the authorities over a week to identify her and notify me of her death, however, the night she died and the first night thereafter, I was woken from deep sleep to hear a voice calling loudly, "Mom!"

Her laughter, her suffering and her gifts were many — and varied. For me, her mother, from the first time she opened her eyes, she unzipped my heart to love and pain and to a life with changes and growth beyond anything I had ever imagined. She demonstrated the ability of a determined person to rise above a dire prognosis of what life could hold for her, of what a person might achieve and what they might give to others. She taught me both to love and to let go. This was her legacy: Trick or Treats? In the end, perhaps a little of both.

You can find strength and hope when faced with the difficult challenges life sometimes surprises us with. When faced with a terrible and terrifying situation, try to remember that negative events sometimes hold deeper meanings. Accept the challenges you are given as an opportunity to learn and grow. Remember to love and forgive yourself as needed at the end of each day. It's all an ongoing learning experience! Every moment offers a new opportunity to rise again.

IGNITE ACTION STEPS

- Start your day with a gratitude practice. Focus on at least three things for which you are grateful and embellish on them. It could be something as simple as having hot water to wash with. Make a gratitude journal to review when things seem dark.

- If you find yourself dealing with a health issue, search the internet for more information. Talk with others who share your concerns. Seek out support groups where you can meet others with similar challenges. Post notices and see if you can create a local group where you can meet in person to share a cup of tea or a hug.

- Meditate on compassion. Take a moment when you wake in the morning or at bedtime to look in a mirror. State your name out loud and remind this person of their qualities, strengths and send them love. Keep going — even if it is painful to accept your own inner beauty. If you are a caregiver or have a caregiver, name that loved one and remind yourself of all the qualities you admire and love in them.

- Get energy treatments or massages. Take a moment in nature to revive. Take time out to watch a comedy or laugh with friends. If you are a caregiver, remember that in order to give, you must take moments to care for yourself, too.

Dianna Delacoeur - United States
Delacoeur Energy Flow Alternative Therapy founder & practitioner;
Reiki Master; T.T. Practitioner; R.N.
delacoeur@att.net

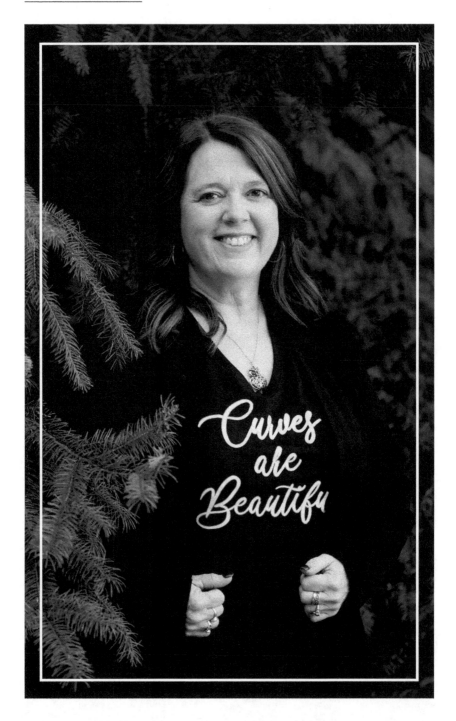

CHARLENE RAY

"Love and celebrate your body; there are so many ways to be beautiful!"

I hope this story will touch your heart. Perhaps you will see yourself in it and be inspired to be kinder toward yourself. I would love for you to transform your negative self-talk into a love and appreciation for the one beautiful body you were given.

BE YOUR OWN KIND OF BEAUTIFUL

This is not the story of losing 50 pounds and living happily ever after, even though it could be. I have lost numerous pounds a number of times in my life. Too many times to count. Instead, this is the story of learning to love the body I have, after many years of suffering. The truth is, this is a story I am still living.

I don't look at my body. Ever. At least not without clothes on. And I only look with clothes on to make sure I don't go out of the house looking ridiculous.

I often imagine that I am the only one this hard on myself. I'll catch my reflection in the mirror and tell myself that my face is just too round. I'll put back that cute sleeveless top I own because someone might look at my flabby arms. I've even been mean enough to call myself names like 'whale, fatso and ugly.' Words I would never use on someone else. Some days I'm great, other days... I can't believe I'm still struggling with this weight. I have a feeling that some of you can relate.

I believe in the importance of body positivity. I am so happy to be living in a time when we can celebrate many ways of being beautiful. I applaud other large-size people for dressing in colorful clothes, walking with confidence and not letting their size stop them from doing the things they want to do in the world. I sometimes wonder if I will ever be that powerful in my own body.

How I think about my body is deeply embedded in my psyche. It started the moment I was born a ten-pound chubby baby. I grew up in a time when 'thin was in.' All my friends knew: the thinner, the better. It was a fatphobic culture. Tiny-waisted Barbie dolls were my childhood companions. Magazines like Seventeen and Cosmo had me wanting to be like the wafer-thin models on their pages. Those magazines showed me just how I should look and what was acceptable. I told myself I was never acceptable.

My mother was the most beautiful, generous, and thoughtful woman I knew. Yet she was obsessed with weight. She wasted far too much of her life energy on diets and worrying about size. I can remember her hiding in the garage to sneak a snack cake before coming into the house to eat a 'respectable' salad for dinner. While others saw her as this wonderfully kind person, she was the most unkind towards herself. She was obsessed with thinness; she started me dieting at the young age of eight. I loved food when I was a child. Dieting was horrifying to my soul and set my body on a course for a metabolic train wreck.

I remember walking into Weight Watchers, as a not-so-little eight-year-old, to get weighed, knowing that I had cheated on my diet that week. The candy, chocolate and deep-dish pizza were just too good to pass up. If I managed to stay the same weight, it was a relief. It was not *great*, but not as shameful as the days my weight was up by a pound or two. And if by chance I lost weight, I was elated. My self-worth was based on the scale and I got on that scale more times a day than I could count.

I allowed the cultural standards to govern my feelings about my body and believed all the things I was told by the adults around me. At age six, I believed the dance teacher who told my mother I was too fat to dance. And the sales clerk at the Sears Department Store who told me to head over to the 'chubby' section where I would find only the ugliest clothes. None of the cute outfits came in my size. Shopping for my wardrobe was an experience to dread. My large-sized godmother worked at Lane Bryant, a plus-size clothing store, and I hated going near it. In those days, clothes for fat girls and fat women were made just to cover the body with no attention to style. There was nothing beautiful for fat girls.

I remember overhearing a conversation between my parents when I was just 10. My father told my mother, he was afraid that I would end up an old maid — a woman who was never acceptable enough to marry — like my godmother.

"Boys don't like fat girls," he said. I was devastated. My father and I adored each other, which made his statements even more crushing to my little heart. My parents were good, loving parents. Had they known I overheard that conversation, they would have been upset, never wanting to hurt me.

Hearing him, I vowed to never eat again. Of course, that vow was followed by a binge on grandma's homemade chocolate chip cookies. When the mean girls at school — and worse, the girls I thought were my friends — chanted derogatory rhymes or squeezed me between the desks, or the cute boy made comments on needing a forklift for me to move, I would come home in tears, feeling absolutely alone. My grandmother always knew how to make me feel better with homemade treats. At my house, food equaled love.

That love was diminished when my father died, despite all the cooking my grandmother did. Homemade bread and pies filled the kitchen as I withdrew and retreated to my room. The grief from losing my father at 13 was intense and I had no one to talk to about it. I was left with a huge hole in my heart. I felt like no one cared about me or understood. I grieved by looking at all the ways I was not perfect. Clearly, if I were a better daughter, he would not have died. I had so much body hatred and my abusive self-talk was both negative and horrible. I never spoke to anyone the way I spoke to myself.

I had been so alone with my pain. I could have turned to my usual comfort foods, but this time, I became an expert calorie counter. I memorized the calorie counting book and knew all the foods that were under 50 calories a serving. On the outside, I put on a happy face. I was a good girl who got good grades, always smiling, always ready to help. I often wondered if, beneath the outside appearance of having it all together, other people were also feeling negativity toward their body and talking meanly to their image in the mirror. My life was forever changed by the death of my father as I internalized the grief. Without anyone to talk to, I decided to become a counselor because of it.

When I got older and lived away from home, my phone conversations with my Mother always started the same: they began with an account of who had gained and lost weight, and what size they were wearing. "Suzie's a size two and she's lost weight. Sally's a bit depressed so she's been gaining weight." This was her way of describing how everyone she knew was doing and feeling. I remember finally saying, "Mom, I can't take it anymore. I don't care how much people weigh. It isn't important to me." She was astonished by that comment and it was followed by a very long silence. It didn't stick. By our next conversation, she was back to sharing everyone's measurement updates.

In my early twenties, during my lowest weight, I still felt imperfect. After checking off another three-hour workout on my calendar and feeling pleased that I had exercised for 28 consecutive days, I looked in the mirror and grabbed what I could squeeze of my nearly flat stomach. I said, in a self-deprecating voice, "You are so fat. I hate you."

Getting into my car to go home, I burst into tears. I was exhausted. The negative self-talk had drained my energy. I could not keep up the daily three-hour workouts at the health club and I could not bear all the time I spent thinking about food, deciding what to eat, and when and how much. My relationship with my husband was suffering. I was as thin as ever, but I was irritable and depressed. I knew something needed to change.

I found a therapist who specialized in eating disorders. Body dysmorphia wasn't even a diagnosis back in the late '80s, perhaps because it was so normal to hate your body and be dissatisfied with it. Therapy and listening to Shad Helmstetter's book *What to Say When You Talk to Yourself* was a good start on my journey to recovery. I made affirmation cards that I read every morning and I listened to a tape of body-affirming messages in the car. Healing was very difficult. I feared gaining weight more than anything. I spent the next few years slowly learning to appreciate and accept my body. This continues to be a difficult and daily practice.

One of my favorite Mary Oliver poems begins with these lines...

> *"You do not have to be good. You do not have to walk on your knees for a hundred miles through the desert repenting. You only have to let the soft animal of your body love what it loves."*

Two months before my Mother died, turning forty-nine, I embarked on a vision quest in Death Valley as a preemptive strike on the grief that was to come. I spent 10 days in the desert doing 24 hours of solo time, fasting from food, people and shelter. I consumed my time with writing, reading poetry and reflecting on my mother's life. I was thinking about how she lived and then what I wanted for my own life. Inspired by the poem, I literally crawled on the desert sands reciting over and over "You do not have to be good.".... "You do not have to be thin." I was trying to convince myself of the truth in those words. That quest gave me the strength to be with my mother in her final days.

With the help of hospice care, I remember helping her change into a clean nightgown just a few hours before she died. She looked down at her body, now very small and wasted, and saw the little round saggy belly and said, "I guess I am never going to have the flat stomach that I wanted." I was astonished. A very long silence followed before she spoke again, "I guess it doesn't matter now." I choked back tears, both for the awareness of her impending death, for the life energy wasted pining away for that elusive flat stomach, and my own wasted life energy, also. It was a transformative moment for me. I realized how you feel about yourself as you are about to leave this world should be surrounded by self-compassion and love towards yourself.

A few years later, my metabolic system betrayed me with a low-grade cancer in my thyroid. I tried many alternative methods to get rid of the thyroid nodule before ultimately deciding on surgery. Surgery was scary, but my biggest fear about the procedure was the possibility of gaining weight after. Looking back, I found this very revealing. Those beliefs about my body ran deep.

Healing from surgery was easy, but I started gaining weight, just as I feared. Because I had learned from my grandmother that food is love and comfort, I ate to feel better. Then, the familiar pattern of dieting began. I increased my exercise. I tried the keto diet, the paleo diet, vegan diet, intermittent fasting, and nothing worked. Eventually, I gave up trying.

Soon, another familiar pattern had reemerged: negative self-talk, body hatred, and self-loathing. I looked in the mirror and called myself fat. Then, I stopped looking in the mirror. I stopped looking at my body. I would have jumped out of it and left it behind if I could have.

On the outside, I did the same thing I did many years before. I tried to dress nicely, I faked confidence at work, I told myself it didn't matter. Then, one day, a client came to see me because she was experiencing anxiety. She hated her body. She loathed herself. She was the age I was when I started the meanness towards my body. I watched this beautiful Being in front of me and listened to her self-talk and self-hatred. It was like looking at a reflection. I could see her beauty and her suffering. When I was her age, I also felt that suffering. Something in me shifted at that moment. I saw what I had been doing all those years to myself. The veil was lifted.

I went home and wept. For her and for the suffering and pain she was in, and for me and all the lost years, the wasted time obsessing over my body and the quest for the elusive flat stomach. I wept for the 10-year-old girl inside me who heard the father she adored say she was going to be an old maid, and that no one likes fat girls.

That evening, I found my old affirmation cards and I read them. I pulled poetry off the shelves and read *Love After Love* by Derek Walcott.

"Peel your own image from the mirror. Sit. Feast on your life."

Amidst the tears that were still flowing, I made a list of what I loved and appreciated about my body. Top of the list was that it created, carried and birthed my amazing son. My body is the only one I have; it is the vessel with which I am able to do the work I am called to do.

After that Ignite moment, I began to dance again. I pulled out the mindful self-compassion materials that I use with clients and used them with myself. I continued to think about good healthy food choices and I also allowed myself to enjoy the foods I love. I bought new clothes that made me feel good and ignored the size on the label. I started following body positive models, influencers and groups on Instagram. I read inspirational and self-affirming poetry every day. I gave gratitude for the body I have been given and thanked it every day for being strong and healthy. I didn't lose a pound through all this, but I felt more powerful.

I am convinced that there is enough power trapped in body loathing and hatred that, if it were freed, it would transform the world. My life journey with learning to accept my body started with birth, got wrapped in grief, and has been my focus ever since. It has been an up-and-down roller-coaster ride of a journey. One I'm still on.

Today, I help others celebrate their bodies. I don't want them to go through what I went through. I help them see their beauty. I teach them about how powerful it is to talk to themselves with kindness and compassion. I help my clients recognize how the culture holds them back and keeps their power small. As they begin to embrace and accept their body in a positive way, it transforms their lives and it is such a blessing to watch that process... to see it radiate from the inside out. It is a gift to watch my clients take back their power and begin to stand for who they are and what they believe.

This is the ongoing journey for many towards health and wellness. It takes courage and self-love to celebrate who we are. Be your own kind of beautiful!

IGNITE ACTION STEPS

- Take a few minutes to reflect on these questions: "How do I really feel about my body?How do my feelings hold me back from living the life I want to be living?" You may wish to write your answers in your journal.

- If you catch yourself saying something hurtful or negative about your body, pause for a moment. Take a deep breath. Notice how it feels to hear those harsh words. Soften your attitude toward your body and say something soothing and loving to yourself. Here are a few examples: "I am here for you.", "I will be more gentle toward you.", "You are beautiful just as you are."

- Make a list of what you love and appreciate about your body. Post your list in a place where you can read it regularly. *Don't skip this one and think you don't have to do it.* Recognizing your own beauty and being reminded of it reinforces those positive messages on the brain.

- In a conversation with a friend or loved one, tell the story of your relationship with your body and what you have learned. Talk about yourself in positive ways from birth to present, including stories and ways that can have more self-compassion. There is healing in sharing your story.

- Name three ways you can celebrate the body you have. For example, I love to dance when no one is looking, put on wonderful lotions after I shower and wear clothes that are comfortable. Say thank you to your body and do one thing to celebrate your beautifulness today!

Charlene Ray - United States
Heart-Centered Mentor, Spiritual Counselor, and Workshop Facilitator
www.charleneray.com
⊙ revcharleneray

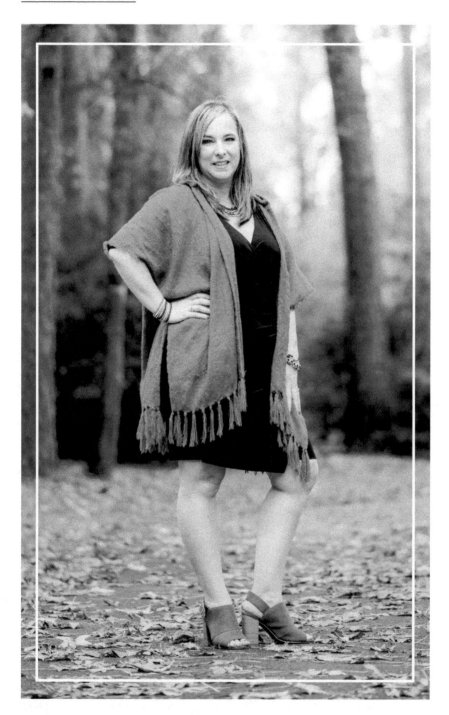

EMILY C. ROSS

"YOU are the Hero of your own story."

Many individuals waste years auditioning other people for the role of Hero in the story that is their life. During that dormant time an inner Hero is waiting to be awakened along with true power and purpose. Trauma can derail people from their true life path, as they become consumed with easing their pain. This chapter is dedicated to individuals in the pursuit of whole-person healing. I am speaking to people who acknowledge the mind-body connection but still do not feel whole. May these pages Ignite a sense of reverence for your soul's path and inspire you to step into the role of Hero in your own story.

SOUL HEALING

When someone you love completes suicide, it creates a chasm that will forever divide your existence into two segments: before the tragedy and the aftermath. For a long time that was the only thing I could be certain about, that my life now had a before and after. It was an uninvited plot twist in an already bad improv that had become the story of my life.

A truth about my mother's life was that nothing was ever easy for her. This was a constant she clung to as she attempted to facilitate her own death. My mother shot herself, no doubt anticipating a quick end to a life she could no longer bear. I can almost hear her mind reasoning that the rifle was sure to be as swift and effective with ending her life as it had been with the many squirrels it had been used to rid the garden of before her. It seemed like a reasonable expectation but what she got instead was a six-week stay in a medical intensive care unit. There her body ultimately gave in to her mind's wish and succumbed to the complications related to her self-inflicted gunshot wound. Her body held on those six weeks, surviving to just minutes before my 37th birthday, in a final effort to be sure to traumatize my meager existence beyond all repair.

Readers who have not survived the suicide of a loved one are likely shuddering and fighting back accusations like selfish and callous, or worse, guessing which stage of grief I am in. The human language lacks the adjectives necessary to describe the vortex of time between when my mother attempted suicide and when she was finally granted the reprieve she sought. I was a silent witness to six of the most physically painful weeks of her already painful existence.

I believe my mother's suicide was the final stop on her lifelong pursuit of healing. Since I can remember, my mother's Soul had been on an epic quest for a reprieve from childhood abuse, chronic trauma and decades of substance use. She endured more trauma than any other human I know and I can empathize that she was tired of her futile attempts to feel better. It is true that she tried many things:

She tried eating organic whole food; she tried eating her feelings. She tried supplements and power foods. She tried restricting her food.

She tried every mind-altering substance she could find; she tried sobriety.

She tried Eye Movement Desensitization and Reprocessing, trauma therapy, hypnosis, talk therapy, Cognitive Behavioral Therapy, self-help books, mental hospitals, medications and multiple 12-step programs.

You name it, she wholeheartedly tried it. She was *that* desperate for a cure to her pain. My mother, like many others, was missing a vital piece. The piece of healing most often overlooked. When a trauma occurs it impacts our Mind, our Body and our Soul. To truly experience healing, we must address each of these areas. There is no other way to true, long-term, whole person healing. If any one of these areas is left unattended, the trauma will continue to seep out into other areas, demanding to be expressed, begging to be acknowledged and healed.

It has become normalized to discuss the mind-body connection because people are now understanding that the food we use to fuel our body impacts our ability to think clearly, our mood and even our emotions. It is well known that the way we talk to ourselves can literally make our body sick. While the mind and body are both very important — what about your Soul? When the Soul is sick, the mind and body suffer as well. We cannot allow our quest for wellness to leave our souls unnurtured and neglected.

True healing must occur on a Soul level as well. This type of healing cannot take place until we are reconnected to a Higher Power. The belief that your Soul must be connected to a Higher Power does not dictate the nature of the relationship your Soul is to have with this said power. The factor necessary for healing is only that the relationship exists. This connection need not follow an organized scripture or a particular doctrine to promote healing. Healing is not contingent on calling your Higher Power by a particular name. It will happen whether you call your Higher Power God, Yahweh, Allah, Jehovah, Buddha, the Universe, Heavenly Father, Jesus, the Holy Spirit or any of the many more names we have given to this source over the centuries.

Healing is not in the names or the rituals; the healing is in the connection to your source. It is in remembering that you are a part of something larger than yourself or your trials; it is in trusting events are guided by a force greater than human understanding. Surrendering to these truths is all that is necessary to initiate the healing process at the Soul level. It is as simple and as complicated as that.

The Soul often gets ignored in the healing process because it is not as easy to monetize and things that are free do not require marketing. We are not constantly bombarded by our need for products and programs to heal our Soul by the media, entrepreneurs or on social media. However, we get blasted by a constant stream of products to heal the body: personal trainers, exercise programs, nutritional products and supplements. They come from multiple sources: ads, friends with multilevel marketing businesses, television, billboards, radio and even on our phones.

Tons of products exist to heal our minds: hundreds of therapy techniques, ketamine treatments, Electroconvulsive Therapy and psychotropic medications offered by a plethora of providers including therapists, social workers, health coaches and psychiatrists. Conversely, connecting the Soul to its source is free, but because humans can not readily profit from it, no need exists to market it. It gets difficult to notice amidst the constant barrage of all the products for sale to help cure our minds and bodies, facilitate their connection and chase the promised healing. The reality is we have come to rely on the media to tell us what we need, and soul healing is consistently left out.

Like many others, my mother did not realize it was her Soul that was tired. Her desperate need to heal her own traumas led to her creating traumas for me, and by the time she completed suicide, my Soul was tired too; that is what generational trauma does. When the pain becomes too much for one human to carry, they pass it down to the next, like handing off a baton in a relay race.

The day she shot herself she handed me the baton of her traumas, which I was then obliged to add to my own. I was instantly heavier with the weight. I did what humans do, joining countless others in my own personal quest to feel peace through healing pain.

No matter how thoroughly life seems to be falling apart, the world is simultaneously beautiful. People love to throw scenarios at me when I declare this, but it is always true. When my mother was clinging to life on a surgical intensive care unit 656 miles away, I could have focused on how tiring it was traveling back and forth, how daunting it was to make medical decisions for my mother or how I did not have family or friends where I lived so I had to bring my school aged children with me on each 70 hour round trip to the hospital.

I do lament those difficult parts of the experience, but I also recall that the hospital was located across the street from the ocean. This offered us breathtaking sunsets and evening walks with the smell of saltwater in the air. Each evening, my daughters and I would enjoy sunset picnics at tables by the beach. They would collect seashells and hunt for hermit crabs. These moments offered us a beautiful reprieve from focusing exclusively on the hard parts of the experience.

I started trying to heal the grief, anger and pain that had become the baton of my trauma by focusing on healing my body first. I lost 70 pounds, ate organic raw wholefoods and raced half marathons. I did not feel better, so I focused on healing my mind. Therapy, yoga and mindfulness practice all helped, yet I still did not feel healed or whole.

I looked better and knew how to meditate, but I still felt tired. I started searching for other things and ironically tried all the quick fixes my mother taught me. Until someone spoke to me about the power of prayer and invited me to church. Reluctantly, I went and quickly I connected with like-minded people who were joyfully living happy, healthy lives. They were healing their trauma by helping others, releasing their heaviness with the lightness of faith.

My past began to make sense and affirmed that 'meaning' exists even in the midst of pain and tragedy. When you give it over and let go, seeing that you cannot change, fix or redo the traumatic experiences but instead uncover the gift entwined in it all, you feel a sense of peace that frees your mind to see the beauty that was hidden in plain view all along. I was able to honor the sadness while simultaneously acknowledging that I am still entitled to be successful, happy and free.

Healing happened for me when I began to nurture my Soul by reconnecting to my Source. For me, this involved re-establishing my relationship with

Heavenly Father through my Savior Jesus Christ. The knowledge that my soul's path is part of a larger plan Ignited in me a faith that inspired deep peace and ended the battle within my soul. This awakened me to the infinite possibility that *He* has an amazing life in store for me.

Nurturing the relationship with my Source heals my soul. And like physical and mental health, healing in this area requires consistency. Just like when not eating healthy and exercising leads to illness, not attending to your spiritual health leads to your soul feeling disconnected, tired and heavy. It is commonly understood that to heal trauma we need to address the ways trauma impacted our body and our mind. What is uncommon is acknowledging that your soul has a component in true, whole-person healing. You can be the exception, living not just your dream, but also your best life, by becoming the *Hero* of your own story. The power is in you to reconnect to Source. Find your passion and purpose by healing Your Soul.

IGNITE ACTION STEPS

So many paths exist to true healing of our body, mind and soul. It is imperative that you attend to each of these areas when healing from trauma but which modality you choose to heal each is what will make your path unique and your journey your own. Use these suggestions only as a guide to access your own intelligence as you revise, revisit, remember and return to your rightful place as the Hero in your own story.

1: Nurture your *Mind* by noticing the collateral beauty

Vigilantly train your mind to notice all that is beautiful in the world, especially when it is difficult. Fortunately for me I had become adept at this by 2017 when Hurricane Harvey flooded my home, killed my farm animals and destroyed literally every material possession I owned. I was over 40 with three children, three dogs, four cats and now homeless. It is doubtful any reasonable human would have criticized me for feeling hopeless, helpless or overwhelmed. I could have given up, tapped out or passed my baton of trauma on to my children.

Instead I got so busy soaking up all the collateral beauty that the event became a profoundly positive turning point for me, and by association, in the lives of my daughters. I wallowed in gratitude for all the ways that people showed up to help us — from prayers and cards to practical items like clothes and money. I could focus on that experience being my lowest point but I had never felt so loved! Instead of passing on the baton of trauma, I showed my children how to find Hope and cling to it. *This is how generational trauma is healed.*

Admittedly, finding the beauty in difficult situations can be challenging. That is why it is imperative to practice this daily. In our house we do this by sharing our favorite parts of the day. If a family member has had a particularly hard day, it is likely I will encourage them to find three or four good parts. They don't know I am training their minds for when tough times come. In fact, they think it is an annoying game their Mother enjoys torturing them with. But I know something they have not learned yet: the more this skill is practiced, the easier it gets. I promise when something potentially life-shattering occurs, you will be grateful to remember to notice what is simultaneously beautiful.

2: Nurture your *Body* with proper nutrition and movement

If you listen to your body it will tell you what it needs: water, nutritious raw whole foods and movement. We know these truths, yet when life gets busy it is easy to choose the convenience of processed food devoid of nutritional value. We eat to assuage feelings rather than to provide the fuel our body needs to do the amazing things we require of it.

You know the right thing to do in this regard: train your mind to make healthy food choices every day. Do not do this with a goal to look any certain way or to see a specific number on a scale. Eat to nourish your body because your body deserves it.

Move your body often. Dance, walk, climb, bounce, cycle, crawl... just move! Running changed my Life. I started out at 170 pounds and a sedentary lifestyle, but over the course of a year I increased my distance, and ultimately ran a half marathon. And then another and another. When I consistently run 7-10 miles a day my body craves healthy food, I get full faster and require fewer calories than when I am sedentary.

3: Nurture your *Soul* by connecting to your source

So many ways exist to connect with your source. Prayer, church, reading religious doctrines, nature, meditation... the list is infinite. My personal practice involves many of these but my favorite way to nurture my connection with Heavenly Father is by consistently living the concept of Karuṇā.

Karuṇā is referred to in Sanskrit, Hinduism, Buddhism and Zen practices.

It translates to 'compassionate action,' which is any act that has the goal of helping others in reducing their suffering. For me, this is how we nurture our Soul healing. An irony of life is that the biggest benefit to helping others heal is that your Soul heals through the process.

Practicing Karuṇā daily can be achieved through small acts of kindness or consistent volunteer efforts. The more you are able to weave this concept into the fabric of how you interact with the world, the more healing you will help others achieve and the more you will benefit yourself.

Emily C. Ross - United States
LPC, Integrative Medicine Provider, Certified Trauma Provider
EmSpiration
life.by.emspiration@gmail.com
f *life.by.emspiration*

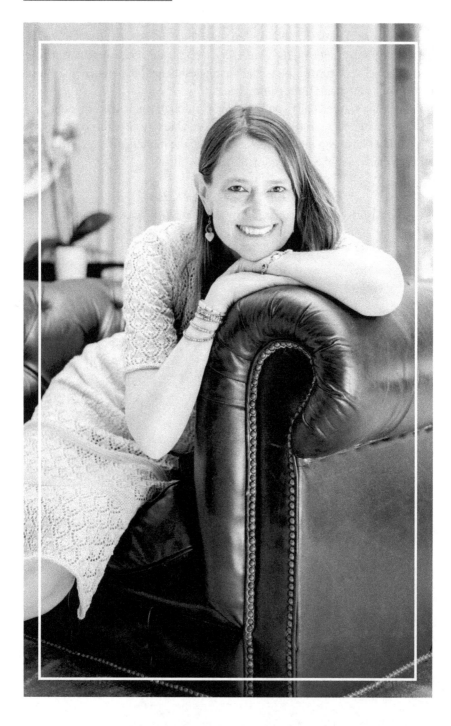

KATARINA AMADORA

"Healing lies within… seek not outside of yourself.
Align body, mind and spirit and you will soar."

My intention is to inspire others to take responsibility for their own health and to educate themselves so that they don't give over their power to anyone outside themselves.

THIS IS YOUR BODY, YOUR LIFE

Remember when you were a kid? That sense of infinite wonder as if any-thing were possible? I fear sometimes that as adults we have robbed our kids of having that same sense of infinite possibility which we enjoyed. We are handing over a world that is dramatically different from the one that we grew up in. I didn't have to worry about inheriting a planet that is ravaged by climate change or the economic disparities which exist today. Back then, there really was a sense that I could be anything I wanted.

I remember my 6th birthday, opening my present to find a doctor's kit. It was made of yellow plastic and it had three bottles of candy pills in the side. It had a plastic stethoscope and microscope as well as a pretend thermometer and syringe. I soon stocked it with all sorts of other things… bandages and real syringes from the doctor's office without the needles. I had so much fun that day. I put one sister to bed and gave her candy pills while I took the other one's temperature. I felt powerful… at last I could make everything better; I wanted to make everyone well. In that moment, I had found my calling. I was going to be a doctor!

Most adults did not take me seriously; after all, kids change their minds all the time. Not me. Any doubt that someone cast my way had the opposite effect; it just made me more determined. I was too stubborn to be dissuaded and my ambition became a badge of honor for me. I was going to be a Doctor.

There was so much in my life that I could not control. Somehow, I think I saw becoming a doctor as a way to take back control. Mom took me to the doctor when I was sick and he would fix me. He would give me a pill or a shot and I would get better. I wanted to be able to do the same thing. I wanted to be able to fix *everyone.*

I think that need to 'fix' others came from my desire to fix my father. He suffered from a mental illness called Schizoaffective Disorder. The most vivid memory from my early childhood was when I was four years old and he unnecessarily shouted at me for bringing my doll downstairs. Petrified, I ran outside to hide among the fragrant Lilies of the Valley beside our house. I still remember what it felt like, hiding beside the chimney, wondering if it was safe to go back inside, waiting for my mom to finally come and find me.

The next day, they took him away and he did not come home for six weeks. When he finally returned, he was different. He was on medication, but this was not the father I had known. Nothing would ever be the same again after that fateful day. Over the years, he relapsed into insanity and paranoia again and again. Each time, he would be taken away. After a while, I wished they would not bring him back. I wanted my mom to divorce him, but she wouldn't. I had no respect for him. He was fat and smoked like a chimney. He smelled bad all the time. I didn't want to be seen with him and certainly did not want to be associated. Even when I was older and he tried to kill my mom, she stayed with him.

I remember that frightening day, hearing the shouting downstairs. My sister and I crept down to see what was going on. As we peered through the crack in the door, we watched my mom attempt to reach the phone to call for help. He ripped the phone from the wall and put his hands around her neck. We ran across the street to our neighbor's house to have them call for help. I am so glad that my mom had the foresight to make that arrangement so someone knew what to do and who to call (and that she had told us where to go).

The doctors certainly could not fix my dad... I don't know why I thought I could. I guess that type of magical thinking is part of childhood. The problem with making life-altering decisions at such a tender age is that I didn't really think about whether these things would make me happy. I believed that achieving my goal would be the answer. I was sure that being a doctor was the solution to my problems. I think I latched onto this goal out of a desire to have some sense of power. I wanted to make a difference. I didn't understand how medicine really worked or the toll that it would take on me, both mentally and physically. I knew about the long hours in the hospital, but nothing prepared me for the reality of what was in store for me as they indoctrinated me into the Western Medical paradigm.

Medical school challenged me in ways that I had not expected. I was always good at learning and assimilating information, but this was so much more than that. There was an interpersonal component which I had not anticipated. Once my clinical years started, the stress mounted. I was constantly being judged and evaluated by each person that I worked with, from the medical student one year ahead of me, to the interns, 2nd and 3rd year residents, the chief resident as well as each attending physician. For each rotation that I did, I could have as many as five to ten evaluations being submitted regarding my performance. If someone did not like me, they had the power to impact the rest of my career by what they wrote in my evaluation. It was like living in an Orwellian 1984 universe where Big Brother was constantly watching over my shoulder and I could never relax. Sleep was often in short supply as being on call could be very busy, yet I always had to be at my best in every moment. I descended into depression for the first time and was started on medication. My worst fears began to materialize… would I be like my dad? Was this genetic blueprint that I carried going to ruin my life? I refused to consider the possibility that I might have Bipolar, yet the possibility plagued my unspoken thoughts. I did not realize that the way that I was eating was contributing to this biochemistry of emotion. I bought into the genetic hypothesis that mental illness was inheritable and I just prayed that I would never become like him.

Like many people, I was being treated with medication with no attention being paid to the underlying cause of my problems. I have since learned that the allopathic tradition of medicine which is predominant in the western world has been heavily influenced by Big Business. In the early part of the 20th century, the 'powers that be' purposefully suppressed other forms of medicine, all but driving the naturopaths and other alternative medicine practitioners out of practice. Since that time, medical education has been heavily influenced by Big Pharma and the biochemical theory of disease… that there is a pill to cure every symptom. There is a lot of money to be made if you find the right medication for the right ailment. This disease-focused model is very profitable, yet it neglects focusing on what people can do to stay well.

The year after I was born, a physician by the name of Ancel Keys was paid by the sugar industry to publish a study blaming fat for the increasing rates of cardiac disease. At that time, evidence was emerging that sugar was contributing to elevated disease rates, and that was bad for business. The industry got a huge bargain. They paid him roughly $50,000 in inflation-adjusted dollars and he published a study where he cherry-picked data from around the world, systematically excluding the information that did not support his desired hypothesis. This is not how science is done. He excluded nearly two thirds of the existing studies and published his analysis blaming saturated fat for heart disease. This was picked up by the American Medical Association (AMA) and promoted around the world as people were encouraged to follow a diet 'low in saturated fats.'

Many stopped eating butter and became worried about consuming too many eggs. They switched to low-fat milk and margarine as supposedly 'healthier' alternatives. We now know that skim milk contains more sugar and boosts the glycemic index higher, and that the switch to margarine was responsible for hundreds of thousands of deaths, due to coronary artery disease. The trans fats in margarine were far more toxic than the saturated fat in butter. Shortly after this, the government stepped in and for the first time in history, put out food guidelines. I remember when the first recommendations came out. I was in second grade. They brought in a chart to teach us about the four Food Groups. We were to eat four servings of fruits and vegetables, four of breads and cereals, three of dairy and two of meat every day. I went home and told Mom how she 'should' be feeding me.

The adoption of these guidelines led to a pronounced increase in the amount of bread and cereals being sold and consumed, and if you look at epidemiology graphs, a whole host of other chronic diseases began to increase in prevalence. There was no scientific data showing that this is the way that we should eat. These recommendations were based on feedback from lobbyists representing the Grocery Manufacturing Association based on what they wanted to sell to the American consumer. As people took these recommendations to heart, they ate more and rates of obesity and disease began to rise. This has cost the lives of countless individuals as the rates of obesity, diabetes, heart disease and other chronic health problems have skyrocketed. We are all part of one of the biggest failed experiments in history without our consent.

By the time I got to medical school, the word was out: margarine was more toxic than butter. I told my mom to switch back. The truth was much slower to get to the general public and margarine and food with trans fats continued to be sold at an alarming rate. Although I learned some of this, nutrition was otherwise barely addressed in medical school. We were told that obesity is bad and caused disease, but we were not given the tools to address this with patients beyond advising them to lose weight. This is not effective when someone is still eating the same toxic diet that caused the problem and is not given the behavioral support to assist them in changing these addictive habits.

I believe that all physicians go into medicine for the right reasons. They want to help people and make a difference. Along the way, their spirit is crushed by the long hours, the indoctrination, always having to be at their best and live up to every expectation. There is so much to learn, and even if they learn everything that is taught, upon graduation, the average physician is still 15 to 20 years behind the most up-to-date research because this is how long it takes for the new findings to make it into the curriculum. If physicians do not do their own research, they continue to practice based on out-of-date assumptions, particularly in the area of how nutrition contributes to the creation of health or disease.

This has been very profitable for Big Pharma. Iatrogenic deaths are among the three top causes of death in America. Physicians are miserable and have the highest rates of depression and suicide compared to any other profession. I know from personal experience how this feels, and the disheartening realization that even if I had the best of intentions, I could not heal someone as their doctor unless they were willing to take action on their own behalf. This is why more and more doctors retire or leave their practice every year.

My personal health transformation began when I read the book *Grain Brain.* This book had a tremendous impact on me as I completely eliminated gluten from my diet and made a few other recommended changes. Those small changes resulted in me dropping nearly 25 pounds in two years. I then enrolled in a program to become a Holistic Health Coach and learned about the power of the mind to create dis-ease; I was able to wean myself off of medicines that I had taken for years.

In all of my years of medical education, I think only four hours were devoted to nutrition and that was merely the pharmacology of vitamins and minerals. There was absolutely nothing regarding the impact of food on your health. This gap in my education was highlighted for me by Eric Edmeades when I participated in the WildFit Challenge. What I learned blew me away. I discovered how to tune into my body, how different foods make me feel and the impact that these foods were having on my well being.

WildFit changed my relationship with food. At that time, I was happy with my weight but I was intrigued by the health benefits it offered. Listening to the videos, I knew that this was the piece I had been missing. The more I dug in, the more it made sense. Things that I had heard but discounted for years finally got through to me because I was feeling the changes in my body.

Following the WildFit program, I felt my body begin to change. Learning more about the dairy industry made the idea of drinking milk less and less appealing. I began to tune into how foods made me feel. It became easier to say "No" to foods that I now knew were not good for me. I no longer doubted the healing power of food. Over the course of the 90-day program, I released another 20 pounds, returning to my high school weight. I had more energy, mental clarity and better regulation over my emotions. The weight has continued to melt away and I've gone from a size 16 to a size 8. In addition, I have healed years of chronic osteoarthritis and my mobility is better than when I was 40. I have reversed my cellular age by 14 years, according to a Telomere test that I took.

I am grateful that I discovered this new path. Changing my diet gave me the body that I had always wanted while the deep introspection and personal growth work transformed my thoughts and my dedication to my new spiritual path, recontextualized my entire life and gave me the perspective to be able to be with whatever arises, even when it is uncomfortable. I now have a whole new outlook and life just keeps getting better.

Maintaining a WildFit lifestyle has become effortless. I just do not see dysfunctional foods as food, therefore, there is no temptation to eat them. When there is something special that I wish to enjoy, I don't feel guilty about it. I know that I can make that choice without cascading into old, unhealthy eating habits. My transformation has been life-changing. I feel a sense of wonder knowing that anything is possible and I want to help others to experience the same transformation. Now I am a WildFit Coach, Certified Hypnotherapist and Tantra instructor. My sizable toolkit allows me to help individuals and couples experience a complete mind-body-spirit transformation.

Much of our suffering, we create for ourselves. Stories and habits that we pick up in childhood can impact our lives throughout our health span. Address the demons in your closet; they may be making you sick. Thoughts that lead to self-sabotage will steal away your healthy years if you don't heal the source of those thoughts. There are many ways to access the subconscious mind — hypnotherapy, somatic modalities, working with plant medicines in therapeutic settings — all can help you put back together the pieces of a fractured psyche. Don't look for your doctor to prescribe a magic pill. It just does not work that way. Take responsibility for your own life, your health, your diet. Taking back your power feels great, and it is the best place to start if you really want to have the healthy, vibrant life that you deserve.

IGNITE ACTION STEPS

What can you do? Ask questions!!! Understand that medicine is as much an art as it is a science. People give away their power to the person in the white coat and they lose their words when the doctor is present. Your doctor, as well intentioned as he or she is, does not know everything. Inform yourself. Write down your list of questions before your appointment because once you are in the office, I promise that you will forget something that you wanted to ask if you don't have it written down. In the profession, we call this the 'White Coat Syndrome.' Your physician wants to be your ally and you can help them help you by being prepared.

Understand that they don't know what they don't know. It is difficult to keep up with all the latest research and there may be things that they are simply unaware of. Educate yourself about the latest information on health and nutrition. Learn about the Microbiome and its impact on health and disease. Listen to medical Summits that come out regularly, paying particular attention to those that cover issues that interest you. Ask questions. Your doctor will thank you. They may even learn something from you.

If your doctor is not open to the conversation and insists on sticking to out-dated recommendations, get a second opinion. It is OK to change physicians. If they are not keeping up on the latest health and nutrition science, and if they are unwilling to learn, then they are outdated. Find someone who is open to the conversation or has training in the area of nutrition. This is your body, your life. You only get to live once!

Hire a health coach, consult with a functional medicine doctor, be your own advocate! You will determine the experience you have in this lifetime and your health is the most important thing in determining how much you enjoy your time on this planet.

Katarina Amadora, MD - United States
Holistic Health and Intimacy Coach
Certified RTT Hypnotist
Certified WildFit Coach
Tantra Facilitator
www.AmadoraTransformations.com

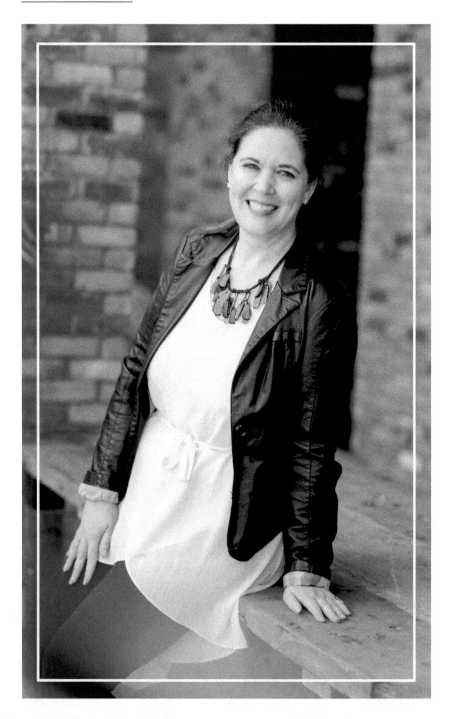

TARA LEHMAN

"I may be shiny, but I ain't new."

Knowing you are flipping through the pages of my story gives me the hope of helping at least one reader understands that the fractures and cracks they see within themselves are not a curse. You will, if you seize the opportunity, highlight the significant, beautiful person you are designed to be.

MY BEAUTIFULLY BROKEN BRAIN

Curled up with hot water beating down on me, I sobbed. Feeling a mix of sadness, anger and indifference, a 20-minute meltdown in the shower was becoming a regular occurrence. I had gotten into the habit of wondering if today was the day I'd sink to my knees in the tub. If I were a betting woman, at best I would break even. It was a total crapshoot.

Let's back up.

At the age of ten, I had my first epileptic seizure. It's impossible to forget. It was the last day of school before spring break started, which of course means excitement to one that young.

It was the end of the day and I'd tossed my backpack over my shoulder, eagerly waiting for the bell to ring. Then, as the tale goes, I frightened the daylights out of my teacher and classmates by collapsing on the floor in a seizure that sent the whole school into a frenzy. One of the kids in my class, whose mother is a nurse, lived across the street and he ran to get her help. Once I was loaded into the ambulance, the first boy I ever kissed ran after it, crying as I was whisked away. It was the first grand romantic gesture in my life and I can't remember it.

Laying in the hospital for a week wasn't so bad. I had fun with the other kids in my unit and used the multiple rolls of quarters my parents brought me to use the payphone so I could call my friends whenever I wanted! It seemed I was fine. No other seizures happened, so everyone hoped that maybe it was just a one-off. That turned out to be wrong. Eventually, I started experiencing two kinds of seizures: the kind where I would collapse in convulsions on the floor every so often and the kind where I would simply blank out for three to five seconds multiple times a day. These second kind were so small that unless you knew me, they were undetectable. But to my great embarrassment, the school saw fit to send the guidance counselor to educate my peers about seizures and what to do if they witnessed me having one.

Ten-year-old me was puzzled by all the attention, but the doctor gave me hope. I can remember sitting in his office, my eyes bright while he explained that if my epilepsy was to go away, it would be before the age of 14. I eagerly awaited that magical age; however, my birthday came and went with no change. I'm now an epileptic veteran having lived with it for over 30 years. I've grown used to it—it's a part of who I am—no different than having my two arms and two legs.

Slowly, I discovered a ritual to ensure my life remained 'almost seizure-free.' It was simple: Take my medication, avoid my triggers and always get enough rest.

Repeat, repeat, repeat.

And the ritual worked... until, one day, it didn't.

My mom was the first to hear of it. She was at my side in the doctor's office as I sat in one of those cold-looking standardized examination rooms that parallelled my mood. I recall it very vividly, despite it happening almost ten years ago. My doctor, a lovely woman whom I really liked and trusted was not beating around the bush. Her eyes were filled with concern as she explained how the child I was carrying had a high chance of being born with conditions such as spina bifida due to my seizure medications; never mind the damage that could be caused if I had a seizure while pregnant. Her words painted very unsettling images in my mind.

I had just found out I was accidentally a few weeks pregnant and she told me what I already knew: If I wanted to become pregnant, I would need to adjust my medications under the supervision of my neurologist ahead of time. Epileptics have healthy children regularly; however, it was too late for that and my chances of delivering a healthy child were lower than we'd like. What struck me in that moment was that I knew having the child was the most selfish thing I could do. Perhaps some people would have taken time to consider their options but not me and I have never regretted feeling that way. Aside from the fact that I had just broken up with the father, who I hoped would never discover I was pregnant, what right did I have to impose this or another condition onto another human being? What right did I have to gamble with the words 'maybe it will be fine'? A parent is there to protect and love her children. In my opinion, I was protecting and loving that child by not risking its future simply because I knew I'd be a great mother. Instead, I made one of the biggest decisions in my life and had my pregnancy terminated, all the while with my father sitting in the waiting room, fully supportive and helping me back home.

This was the pivotal experience required for me to truly understand that epilepsy had the power to impose serious, heart-breaking limitations on me. Of course, I had already been living within the boundaries of what I knew I could and couldn't do; for instance, driving is off-limits for me, but more boundaries suddenly became amplified. They became wider, longer,and louder... and I had to be okay with that.

Now, back to the bathtub...

My body had been sneaky. After almost two years seizure free, I made the mistake of thinking everything was fine and, therefore, didn't get the bloodwork done to ensure my medication levels were as they should be. As a result, my medication levels slowly dropped without my realizing it, which ultimately pushed me to a hard stop. Hard enough to make me collapse in seizures and unconsciousness twice in one day, which had never happened before.

The first one was on the couch, which wasn't so bad since I had a soft place to land. I wasn't so lucky on the second round. That's when I fell in the kitchen where there's all kinds of cupboards and a kitchen island for my head to bounce off of, over and over. These twin seizures gifted me with a concussion bad enough to keep me indoors for the better part of the next three months. My partner tells the story of how I had been drinking coffee during one of the seizures and spilled it all over myself. When he pointed it out to me afterwards, I argued that I hadn't spilled a drop, despite staring down at my coffee-soaked robe. Funny what the brain chooses to see — or in this case, not see — when it's recovering from trauma.

After that, my new normal began. Things like being around three or four people suddenly seemed overwhelming. Within 15 minutes of walking into one of my favorite restaurants, hearing the everyday restaurant sounds made me run to the parking lot in tears. Clearly, my doctor had meant it when she said I needed sensory deprivation. Luckily, I work in a wellness center with amazing healers and was surrounded by their love and understanding, like a great big hug telling me I was doing exactly what I needed to be doing. I spent my days rotating ice packs and heating pads. Making baked goods for everyone became my specialty since I wasn't allowed to use my computer, watch TV, text or read books with small lettering. Occasionally I ignored that advice for the sake of my sanity, and I would get on my computer, setting a 10-minute alarm as my screen time limit.

But let's be honest...

Despite being in my 40s, moms are still moms and mine kept a strict eye on me to make sure I did what I was told. Against my insistence that she didn't need to fly across the country to take care of me, she and my partner conspired behind my back and she appeared on my doorstep. She was determined to take me to any appointments needed and that's all there was to it. It was a rough way to bring the three of us together, but living on opposite sides of the country as we did had made it difficult for her to get to know my partner and it was a great excuse for her to survey my home-front.

The only time I left the house was for my countless massage, physio, craniosacral and acupuncture treatments. Turns out that I am totally capable of falling asleep and drooling on my pillow with needles stuck in my back. I'm certain that all these modalities combined sped up my healing time by months. I was like Humpty Dumpty who fell off the wall, but all of the King's horses and all the King's men succeeded this time and put me back together again!

Until my broken brain healed, it felt like wires were crossing all fuzzy-like where they shouldn't. I felt like I was short-circuiting; two plus two equaled five, kind of thing. I often cried for what seemed like no reason at all, typically in the shower. In hindsight, it's for the best that I cried there as much as I did because it saved a lot of tissue boxes. The water would wash away the salty tears while my partner, mystified, would periodically pop his head in to see if he could help, which he couldn't. These moments were often followed by speedy text messages to my Naturopathic Doctor asking if these meltdowns were normal. Thankfully, she said yes, that the crying was a sign of me getting better.

Looking back, I'm certain some of those tears weren't just because I was concussed. I had been lucky with seizures in the past, if you call faceplanting into a fire hydrant lucky. You just never know when or where a seizure is going to occur and my tears were equally about how my epilepsy hadn't been given the respect it needed, how that situation could have been deadly.

When people preach about how 'anything is possible' and what we can do is simply 'limited only by our dreams,' I beg to differ. They claim if we throw our intentions into the Universe, all will be well. I know some of you may completely disagree and think me a Negative Nellie, and that's fine. My take is simply that if we all had our way, life would be filled with puppies and unicorns running around our flowery gardens. We'd all have a pot o' gold and never have to work long hours to keep the lights on, all while feeling confident and loved 24/7 with rainbows coming out of our arses. Everybody would be healthy. Nobody would refuse to hire you because of your medical condition. Nobody would be like me where, overnight, I went from being a straight-A student to barely passing. I have kept report cards where my teachers wrote they weren't going to grade me since they knew it wasn't my fault that I suddenly couldn't focus and learn the material as quickly as I had in my pre-seizure days. I mean, really... Is it terribly surprising that one doesn't make the honor roll when they're busy blanking out ten times a day? So, no. Not everything is possible in my mind.

Life presents us all with limitations and the beauty of it is that you can learn to play the hand of cards you've been dealt. That's why I tell my neurologist that I feel I have the luckiest form of epilepsy. At first, he was taken aback by my words, until I explained that why else would I choose to look at it any other way? I'm not staring brain surgery in the eye. I'm able to lead a fulfilling life. I'm not one of those epileptics who can't be left alone for fear of hurting themselves, or who find it difficult to hold down jobs and relationships due to how much they seize.

However, that doesn't mean I never struggle with accepting and living with these and other limitations imposed on me. At the time of writing this, I'm in the midst of deciding whether or not to switch medications. With countless pills taken over 30 plus years, I'm aware of the havoc they wreak on my insides and I've discovered what I'll call a cleaner medication which would be easier on my organs and possibly stop my seizures altogether.

I've learned, however, that my life is no longer about chasing a seizure-free life; it's about balance. No neurologist or family member can help me make that decision. They aren't the ones who have repeatedly woken up wondering where they are, unable to move without cringing. They aren't the ones who feel guilty asking someone to drive them somewhere. Nor are they the ones crying in the bathtub over the adventures they have to say no to. It's my responsibility to make a choice.

I've often wondered what life would be like if I wasn't epileptic. It's a trap every single person dealing with a chronic condition falls into. We ask ourselves: Would my better-behaved electrical energy make my personality so very different? I wonder… Would I feel smarter? Lose my creative side? Without my epilepsy, would I have attracted the same type of people into my life?

Given our brain has millions of cells controlling the way we think, move and feel, I think it is impossible to be the same person I am without my epilepsy. The hand of cards I have been dealt is not what I would have chosen, but it has taught me much and shaped who I am. And I like who I am. I have all that I need. Sure, my life is snagged in such a way that I can't do all of the things I'd like to, but whose isn't?

Life is divided by things we can and can't control. So, I focus on what I know to be true: epilepsy doesn't need to be the deciding factor in all that I do. Instead, it is meant to be taken into consideration with every decision made, which means not being stupid and arrogant enough to think I know my body better than it does. My body came with its own template, stamped with rules that I do not have the luxury of breaking.

According to the World Health Organization (WHO), around 50 million people worldwide have epilepsy, making it one of the most common neurological diseases. The unfortunate part of that is the stigma surrounding epilepsy can often be more difficult to overcome than the seizures themselves. This can manifest in discouraging people with symptoms to get diagnosed, so as to avoid becoming identified with it.

I don't think of epilepsy as a disease. Clearly it is — WHO says so and, therefore, I can't argue — but at this point, I just look at it as a lifestyle. Luckily, I live in a country where there is acceptance of epilepsy — not to be confused with the understanding of it — and I realize that not all epileptics worldwide have that privilege. In both China and India, epilepsy is viewed as a reason for prohibiting marriages. If something as common as epilepsy is looked upon this way, how many other medical conditions are categorized the same way?

We all have limitations in one way or another, and that's okay. When faced with something out of your control, rest assured you can make the best life with what you do have. You can choose to focus on what you know to be true and real. Celebrate the things that make your days the best days ever. Educate others whenever you can, and when you fall, always get back up. Literally.

FELICE MARANO

"Grant yourself the right to be a unique gift to the world."

My intention is to positively transform the existing paradigm about people living with HIV. To give endless hope and strength to millions of people suffering because of a tough diagnosis made even harder by prejudices, misconceptions and ignorance. My profound desire is for my story to touch the souls of those suffering from mental health problems and life changing diseases — regardless of their nature. I strongly aspire to inspire a liberating path through the realization that we are the masters, the creators and the healers of our own spiritual, physical and mental lives.

DISRUPTIVE REFLECTIONS ABOUT LIFE WITH HIV

Everybody has a story to share — an Ignite moment, that exact second there is no other perception than fire burning within bones against any layer of the human flesh. Every human *is* a story. What we share as living creatures is a deep need to connect, speak loud our truth. It is that penetrating response controlling the inner self, paralyzing every cell of the body, transforming tragedy into acceptance, surrender into fear. Fear of not being able to open up, of ending completely naked, unarmed, exposed to the unknown. So scared and yet so potentially authentic, ready to let go of blockages and restrictions. Fear that turns one dull and yet so powerfully wise at the same time. Brave enough to face life-changing actions, sage enough to offer life the opportunity to progress. Allowing the Self the complete right to be and to exist — the right to be visible.

My story would probably start with the word *invisibility*. Hidden. That disgusting feeling of carrying something society has been rejecting for generations. Not purely a disease, but a combination of stigma and prejudices shouldered by the body. A diverse mixture of horrible stories and narratives.

I believe, it has never been easy to manifest in society as a man living with HIV. To carry within every cell a virus that is not merely devouring every part of the immune system but also consuming every aspect of social connections, family, friends and professional life. A virus that slowly devours every part of the physical, mental and spiritual nature — every single aspect of a living person — until the very last moment when one has no other choice than to rest in peace.

From the very first moment I discovered being HIV positive myself, those were the dramatic thoughts I had in mind. My only references about the HIV virus until then were negative ones. Experiencing early stigma and rejection made me realize that, no matter how far science has gone, there is still much to do in terms of cultural beliefs to help and support people living with HIV, family members and the overall society to deal with a situation that has long been unspoken, left on the side.

This could be my story, a piece of me — my truth to share loud and proud. The intimate story of a young Italian man with the unstoppable desire for traveling the world. The life of a person who fought his entire life to get the best grades at school, the best positions at work, the highest recognitions in every sphere. This honestly is my personal story, but it could be yours — no matter the color of the skin, your country of origin or sexual orientation. No matter if you are in complete health or dealing with a dramatic illness. Regardless of the intense process you are facing right now, life is only manifesting itself to give us opportunities to grow, lessons to absorb and experiences to overcome.

Throwing back to the diagnosis day, it would have seemed impossible to handle such a process if I only focused on the negative aspects of my new condition, still feeling so young and full of life yet a victim of such a dangerous virus. No matter how hard it seemed to deal with such a pain in a small village in Italy, I definitely chose life over death. To empower love, instead of ignorance. To embrace openness over oppression, understanding instead of building up walls – to stand still over running away.

The very first days were extremely painful. I was completely dominated by fear and confusion. Relying on the hospital and its doctors seemed the most adequate way out. Convention, panic and rationality made me approach Western science. To accept the sole solution of taking a huge pill every day, at the same time and for the rest of my life.

I was paralyzed. I could not believe I had to face such a dramatic diagnosis and process toxic reflections at night before sleeping, knowing the effects of a drug would gradually invade my brain. Shaping thoughts that never belonged to me—the insidious desire of ending life. The impossibility of differentiating fantasy from reality, present from past — of throwing a line between real life and illusions of the mind, spending hours lying on a bed, completely numb. Unable to smile, unable to breathe, unable to be. I could never deny modern science or be ungrateful for the development of the last decades, the privilege of taking only one single pill per day — not 10 or 20. Or having easy access to a pharmacological treatment and to a complete regular life, able to live fully for years to come. How could I deny being fortunate to become undetectable in only a few weeks? Thus unable to transmit the virus to other people — as researchers have successfully proved in the last years. A milestone in the evolution of the HIV cure.

Gratefulness and openness, therefore, were some of the most important sentiments I allowed after the initial breakdown. They were not enough, however. Not for me, not the two of them alone. I felt something was missing. Aspects and spheres of personal life were not considered. My emotions completely ignored. My energies forgotten. My spiritual life never taken into account, not even superficially considered.

As a result, my inner desire to be much more than just a number or statistic, more than just profit for a pharmaceutical company or a patient for a hospital rapidly emerged. I intuitively felt a need to open up to the world. Speak loud my condition, share my story, give myself the opportunity to *exist*. Regardless of how hard it is for the majority to face disease, suicide or depression. To face the constant, massive fear I still wear on my skin every day.

After a decade of intense travels and experiences around the world, the sanest path to freedom and wellness was allowing my intuition to emerge. Allowing the strong desire to stay. The urgent need to stop exploring the outside world and give myself the chance to explore the inner universe. To stand still. To conceive, shape and reinvent my vision of life and death, health and illness. The way out of a lifelong disease was empowering some of the most powerful tools the human race has been provided with: self-healing and meditation.

In the past 10 years, I have been a diligent yoga practitioner, despite where I was in the world or my main occupation. It took me a long time and a hard condition to realize that listening to myself and uniting soul with body were the best investments I could make. As for any investment, it was time to take advantage of it.

Once I had accepted shame, depression and an inability to be in social situations comfortably, I intuitively decided to sit in front of a white wall, prepare my body, in a comfortable position, connect to my breath and enter a deep status of meditation. I would spontaneously approach this method every day for many hours. In different moments of the day. For the entire day, if needed. I would spend long periods of time feeling my inner energies, perceiving blocks and barriers. I would recognize limiting beliefs and overcome them, gratefully creating a solid connection with my body, my tissues and organs. Feeling them, touching them, liberating them.

No matter how hard it was to handle friends, family and society, I was finally finding the way out from stigma, depression and loneliness. The way out from the pain society was indirectly injecting into me but, most importantly, the distress I was deliberately letting society cause me. The silence gave me direct access to the information I have always stored in my brain. Stories, notions and beliefs I have collected around the world interacting with some of the most brilliant humans on earth. Mental heritage we all have access to simply by experiencing being human. I was finally able to realize life did not end at all. Existence was knocking at my door with all its energy and intention, reminding me how powerful people are for not just being able to radically change any condition but to embrace difficulty as an opportunity to start from scratch. To live once again — from zero. A new person, a completely diverse human being — just stronger, wiser and so important to our society for creating precious transformations. I was given a second opportunity. The chance to build up existence according to my own rules.

The virus did not only offer me the chance to play according to my rules and feel entitled to live life according to my philosophy. It did much more. Illness placed me in direct contact with the perception of death. The violent thought that keeps coming back every hour and every minute, reminding that creation — the way we usually perceive it — could be completely over in a second. A tiny minute, a simple response... and one is gone. Gone from human life — forever.

Previously, I could have perceived everything falling apart, the entire universe at war against me — and I definitely did. I cried, days and nights. Suddenly, it was only me, a so-called disease and I — a radically new being and the uncommon way of approaching reality. I allowed myself to not just be the strongest man in the room, able to spread firmness and power, but the one finally capable of letting go. Able to show up in my own vulnerability. Realizing the relevance of placing first the need to cry and be transparent.

Open and real, rather than compelled to block energies and feed sickness. Illness releases suffering at first. It also offers plenty of power, the holy occasion of not receiving the flow of life passively, but conversely, to take an active part in the sacred process of creation. We are given the fortune to become the creator of our own life, every aspect of it. Our path, our story — and the one linking us to others. We actively start producing life and being life itself the moment we merge with the concept of death. The second we have nothing to lose anymore, we are finally given the sacred possibility to *Be*. To manifest ourselves — as a whole.

Slowly shaping my story, I pursued the need to look for other information, another specialist and the best possible way to treat my precious self. I observed many doctors stuck behind a medical desk, unable to offer practical possibilities, sick and tired of tackling new ways of dealing with illnesses or pain. I wondered how can we all be treated so superficially? Just an average, a file number? Strengthening my belief that in order to maintain health, in modern society, we need to reawaken that deep connection with our own intuition. That powerful force that makes one realize how unique every person is, in their own shape, needs, strengths and fragilities.

The last year truly revealed some powerful realizations. They are the main reason I am here sharing a story. Holding the right to expose something I have been hiding for a long time. Offering illness the right to be unveiled. To be treated for what it really is — separate from judgments and toxic opinions, away from fear. Not treating it as a thing to be ashamed of and to keep it taboo, paralyzed from heavy judgments and stigma that I fear. On the contrary, it is offering the more precious right to focus on a powerful healing process. The possibility to purely show and manifest a condition that deserves healing energy. Giving it the right to exist and absorb curative vibrancies.

I offer permission to my HIV virus to become something real, not something to be denied. Something, instead, to carry in the body proudly — exercising surrender. Not fighting against and being able to integrate any sphere of the complex human being. Strengths and weaknesses, health and illness. To leave cultural concepts behind to transcend duality and expand reality, and any resistance, war or fight. Rather, allowing the body the right to exist and be strong and take responsibility for its sacred nature.

The most powerful thing behind any story, I realize, may not be the story itself. Not the storyteller or the soul behind it. My life is not about myself. It is not about the present, neither about the future. Rather, it is about honoring the millions of people who died years before, the millions of lives that never got a chance to raise their voice — to have a voice. It is about those not able to know the reason of their death, the ones unable to get a cure, a second chance — the opportunity to live the miracle. It is about those brothers and sisters not dying from the illness today but from the stigma and prejudice associated with people living with HIV, the shameful tragedy induced by other humans. Thus inviting us all — no one excluded — to reflect on what humanity really implies.

My words were born to be a disruptive call to existence over the limiting concepts of life and death. An invitation to value the potential humans have to heal not only bodies and spirits but a past of barbarity, tragedy and violence. An invitation to spread the power of releasing true love and healing energy towards any kind of illness and condition in the present moment to cure the past. Giving ourselves, as a species, the opportunity to transform existing paradigms and rewrite the present — to design new history. Endless other opportunities to inspire the future and Ignite millions of people's lives.

Discovering my HIV positive status opened up space for reflections I would not have easily generated before. Firmly realizing we all are in charge of our own health. No matter social condition or personal beliefs, one must always choose to be an advocate for their own health. The sage and the rebel, valuing science and yet not taking for granted every doctor's prognosis, every hospital decision or every stranger's opinion. Liberating healing energies. Honoring sacred intellect. Allowing the miracle to happen.

We should find our own answers and ask the most legitimate questions. We should grant ourselves the right to be our own healer. To be the most important essence, able to feel and scan every microscopic cell of the body, every atom of it. You are the only one entitled to have deep connections with personal reality and needs — with the result of what your mind, body and soul combined can actually do. It is such a powerful realization and a huge responsibility to trust your healing nature, to grant yourself the right to be a unique gift to the world.

Ignite Action Steps

Silence gave me the opportunity to access profound knowledge, reflections and tools to deal with my body, spirit and soul. Before you take any practice, theory or healing process for granted, I invite you to access the most profound essence of the entire existence: your inner Self. Be in presence of the absolute and give yourself permission to manifest and to stand still.

1. **Preparation.** Sit in a comfortable position — back supported, head free. Observe your breathing — literally just observe. It may be calm or very fast. You may have some difficulties in breathing. In this phase, you are only acknowledging it. No need to change anything. You do not want to create any resistance. Just allow yourself to be.

2. **Conscious breathing.** Take an active part in the breathing process. Start only using your nostrils. Inhale for two seconds and exhale for four. The aim is to double the exhalation to calm the nerve connecting the brain with the body. Keep the cycle going for five times or more.

3. **Grateful silence.** It is time to give yourself permission to merge with the rising silence. It may be complicated at first to focus on silence, thus I invite you to keep in mind one of the most powerful mantras: *thank you.* Start hearing the words slowly appearing at the background of your mind. Thank you! Thank you! Notice I wrote hearing it, versus saying it. Slowly start perceiving the mantra becoming softer and fainter until disappearing completely. Thoughts will appear and concerns will rise. Don't judge — it is part of the ongoing process. Do not even fight against this natural flow. The one and only thing you must do at every perceived distraction is to go back to the words. Thank you! Thank you! Let the body do the work for you.

4. **Listen and connect.** Slowly come out of the silence. Give yourself the needed time. Make a deep inhalation and start perceiving your body once again. Enjoy as much time as you need to focus on your physical, emotional or spiritual body. Guide your intuition to perform any instinctive movement or spontaneous healing practice. Use this time to access profound information or feelings you may hold into your precious self. This is the moment to unlock your unique potential. Observe and make a journal of your feelings. Practice every day for about three months, until it becomes a habit.

Spread your gift to the world.

Felice Marano - Italy
Yoga Therapist, Life Coach & Business Innovator
felicemarano@gmail.com
🄵 *hello.felicemarano*
🄾 *felicemarano_*

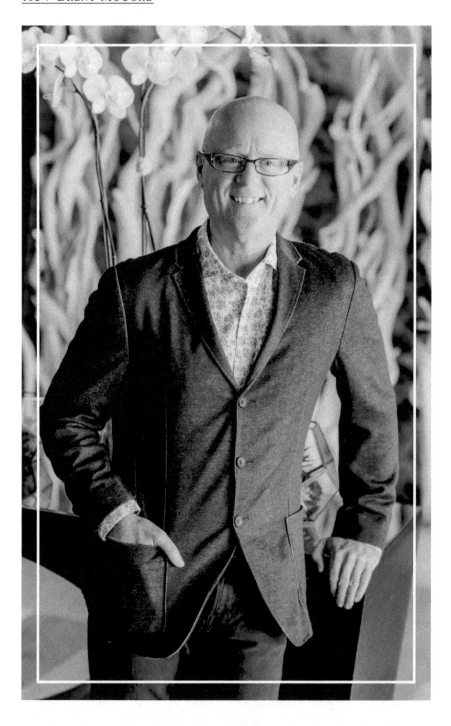

BRENT MCCORD

"Your best life is right in front of you; are you ready to meet it?"

My mission is to empower and ignite your fire and passion for your own accelerated journey of self-care, one that encourages you to make Health and Wellness your #1 Priority. I'm talking about taking personal responsibility for your physical, mental, emotional and spiritual well-being. My intention is to inspire you through my story, the challenges and wake-up calls, the changes and choices I made that raised my health and baseline of resilience. My wish is that you, too, can then design, create and enjoy the life you deserve.

BE YOUR OWN HERO!

Adversity doesn't discriminate. Many of us will face various challenges, grief and hardships. We all can have fears and experience anxiety, stress, overwhelm, addictions, health concerns and more. However, we also have the opportunity to not just survive but thrive!

When I was young, my Mum used to say, "Your health and happiness are everything, more important than money." My father would likely pipe in, "And money doesn't buy happiness either." My Dad was always worried about money. I got a wooden spoon to try and straighten my teeth instead of braces, and played soccer with Reader's Digest books taped under my socks instead of shin pads. He did help me buy my first car and as a family we actually were happy.

I was the oldest of three. My sister, brother and I got along famously and still do. We moved around a lot and ended up in the city of Toronto — what some would consider the 'center of the universe' in Canada — just as I started high school. Dad started working early in life. When he was seven, his alcoholic father left the family. Dad was hard on himself and also pretty hard on me, and I worked at trying to please him. I know he just wanted me to do well and avoid some of his struggles, and it's taken me years to try and overcome my perfectionist tendencies.

My mother was the rock in the family, so loving and supportive to all us kids. She was my #1 fan. She extended her intuition and kindness to her many friends and was adored by all of ours. In high school, I worked nights and weekends, and odd jobs in summer. I tried university for a year but wanted to get out and make money, so I started a career with the leading drug store chain in Canada.

I climbed the ladder while moving back and forth between Toronto in the east and Vancouver and Seattle in the west. I spent my 20s and 30s living on the West Coast and it suited my lifestyle. I loved skiing, golf and sailing, many times doing all three on the same weekend. Eventually I got the call to transfer back to Toronto and, being Power of Attorney for my aging parents, I thought it made sense. Little did I know how quickly my intuition would manifest.

I worked hard, played hard and traveled extensively to the United States and Asia to see suppliers and attend trade shows...Vegas 50 times! Front row tickets to sporting events, luxury boxes, dinners out all expenses paid... there was a lot of VIP treatment. I enjoyed it and it was a great experience... until it wasn't. After 20 plus years, the long hours, late nights, terrible food habits and drinking took its toll.

Being a bit of a rebel, I struggled with the politics and the 'BS' in corporate. I watched my boss get fired after 25 years and won't soon forget watching him walk out of his office with nothing but a small brown box and no watch!

Screw it. I needed a change, some freedom and a new adventure.Time to start building my own business and paying more attention to my health. Time to become the CEO of my own life. I took the leap and left corporate. People thought I was crazy! It was exhilarating to be self-employed in sales, consulting and being my own boss. The financial uncertainty was stressful and I reinvented myself many times over the years. Some failures and lots of wins.

I'd always been a gym rat and stayed in pretty good shape, but I worked out in the early evenings and ate late. I needed some new routines and better nutrition. I decided to challenge my belief that I wasn't a morning person. I started working out in the mornings, got out in the fresh air and nature and started to eat well. I bought more fruits and vegetables, made smoothies, took a few supplements and minimized processed foods. I started feeling better right away.

Early into my entrepreneurial journey, my father was having prostate issues and was diagnosed with clinical depression. Mum was having trouble coping and he ended up in the hospital constipated, delirious and going from 160 pounds to 110 within weeks. I made the extremely hard decision to OK electric shock treatment and it saved his life.

I sold their house and bought them a condo in an assisted living community. For a few years, it was good, but then Mum's health began to decline, starting with forgetfulness. Then there were the incidents. Mum burnt her hand on the stove and my heart sank when she didn't recognize me when I picked her up at the hairdresser's one day. The ultimate crush was when she burst into tears at the psychiatrist's office when asked to spell 'world' backwards and she couldn't. She had full-blown Alzhiemers. Devastating!

Mum went into long term care. When she realized we were leaving her there, she tried to crawl out of her bedroom window. Dad started having falls, and was hospitalized for five months twice, so we moved him into a private residence. My brother and sister helped, but they both had 9-5 jobs so most of the heavy lifting over the years fell to me, commuting back and forth between cities many times a week caring for them. It was stressful for all of us and the emotional labor was exhausting for me. I was trying to be strong, showing no weakness, or emotion because that is how I was brought up.

Struggling with my business and relationship, drinking became part of my coping strategy. I had stress, anxiety, road rage; I felt frustrated and angry. I had to get real. I took a hard look at myself and realized I don't like who I've become. This isn't me. I had always been happy and lived on 'the summer side of life,' but now I was miserable. How the hell was I going to get out of this awful state? It was an Ignite moment.

I realized I could not allow this state of being to continue. It was spilling into all areas of my life and I needed to gain control over it. In my Ignite moment, I realized that life is short. I spent all that time in doctors' offices, hospitals and long term care facilities watching not only my parents but so many others in poor health, losing their dignity, so many with no family caring for them. The main regret of folks in their later years is they didn't live fully and have the courage to follow their dreams. My father was one of them. Good grief, I decided, this is not how I want to go out.

I did yoga at my gym to augment my fitness routine and I knew there was more to explore like mindfulness, meditation and breathwork. I started listen-ing to Deepak Chopra and Wayne Dyer, which had a huge spiritual impact on me. I went many times to an ashram in the Bahamas. All vegetarian meals, no alcohol and lots of yoga, meditation, spiritual learnings and amazing guest speakers. I realized that yoga wasn't something you do but a way of life. They sure don't teach you this stuff in school. It was a game-changer for me. My mindfulness and meditation practice was built around finding compassion, forgiveness and finding grace through gratitude. You have to choose to be happy. Being happier helped me in working and interacting with all the people along the care-giving experience.

Now that I had it back in my own life, I could spread a little joy. I gave up being a victim in this nightmare of watching my parents go through this devastating decline. I went deep within myself and started to realize that all this heartbreak was necessary. It's hard to be conscious and aware when you are consumed by negative emotions. I became less reactive and raised my emotional IQ.

Mum passed at age 79. We had the whole family over to see her on a Friday night. She hadn't eaten or drank for over a week. She lay in bed not moving or speaking, but I know she knew we were there. The grandkids were in tears. I finally went out in the hall and had my first good cry. Shortly after that, everyone left. As I was walking out the door, I thought, "Damn, I'm going to be glad to see the back of this place." In that moment, intuition kicked in and I felt she was going to pass that night. I returned to her room and lay beside her. Almost immediately, I felt her arm come around to comfort me. I couldn't believe it. It was such a gift. She passed at 3AM; God bless her. We had a wonderful celebration of life for Mum with hundreds of her friends.

The months following, I was sad but more relieved she had passed, and I began feeling somewhat guilty. I read an article by someone who experienced the same thing, reminding me that I had actually been grieving losing her for several years. Boy, that saved me! It stopped me from being so hard on myself and made caring for my father easier going forward. Four years later, we moved Dad to long term care and he passed nine months later at 87, completely bedridden, miserable and ready to let go. I told him how much we loved and appreciated him the night before he died.

As part of my yearly checkups, I was getting a PSA blood test, a marker for potential prostate cancer. Most men have some cancer in their prostate but they are more likely to die of something else. This PSA test is not an exact science, in fact, many of the medical associations do not recommend it anymore because of over-treatment causing many men substantial side effects like incontinence and erectile dysfunction. My PSA began rising a few points and right away my urologist wanted to do a biopsy. I have done hundreds of hours of research on every aspect of it and did not elect to do the biopsy. I can understand why many men get them because cancer is a scary word and they just want to know. But there can be complications and I know I don't want surgery or radiation so I thought, "I'll wait." I explored other integrative medicines like an herbalist, naturopathic oncologist, as well as supplements and nutritional considerations. Also, I discovered cancer is only 5 percent hereditary and more likely due to poor lifestyle choices. Who knew?

I had a CT and bone scans to make sure nothing had gotten outside the prostate and it hadn't. A CT scan is as much radiation as 200 chest x-rays so I didn't make the decision lightly. I had a prostate MRI and that found a few suspicious looking lesions that were likely cancer. The radiologist said they would have never found these lesions with the random 12 core needle biopsy because of where they were located. That was extremely validating for me. The urologists were furious that I had gotten that MRI without having a biopsy first. "That's not the way we do things," they told me. "Hmmmm, well that's the way I do things," I replied and we parted ways.

Boom, Ignite wakeup call again! It was time to go full out. I was convinced it's all related to my lifestyle. I managed stress to an even better level, avoided the sugar cancer loves and juiced even more. I identified supplements that may target cancer cells, some specific to the prostate. I reduced meat consumption, only grass-fed beef, organic chicken and wild sockeye salmon. I established detox strategies and became a label reader. I could go on, but you get the point. Yes, it's more expensive, but what is your health and life worth?

I finally found an awesome Uro-Oncology clinic to work with. They believe in MRI vs. biopsy and are fine with me refusing radiation or surgery and exploring new focal therapy ablation (which is finally becoming accepted after many years in trials). It is a tissue-sparing high-heat laser where they blast the tumor, much like what is happening with breast cancer treatments, and it dramatically reduces those dreaded side effects from like 75 percent to 10.

Last year, I discovered I had two spots of early-stage melanoma, one on the top of my head and one on the side of my nose. Great, more cancer! They wanted to do surgery on both, but I asked myself if that was the right choice for me? I got the one on my scalp done, but the nose surgery is invasive and disfiguring, so I asked the surgeon about a new cream I'd discovered on trial in Australia. He said he couldn't recommend it. My dermatologist said he'd never heard of it working for melanoma but reluctantly wrote me a prescription. My lesion was gone in three months.

This health and wellness journey has led me down a path of serious personal growth and a quest to live and reach my full potential. I have collaborated with a global education company that challenges your limiting beliefs and encourages you to become extraordinary in every way. I love the frequent travel and being part of several like-minded communities with so many amazing people. I have learned to honor more of my feminine energy by observing how supportive all these conscious women are to each other. #lifeisgood is my favorite hashtag.

I'm not a physician, and by any means giving medical advice. I'm just saying what I've learned or done, what's worked for me and how I've responded to challenges in my life. I encourage you to take responsibility for the path of your life by designing and creating your own health and wellness plan. As they say on the airplane, "put your own mask on first." Fill your own cup and you will be of even greater service to others.

IGNITE ACTION STEPS

Your health and wellness should be a life-long pursuit and commitment. Here's my morning routine. Up at 6 AM. Make bed. Brush teeth. Drink 20 oz of spring water. Meditate 10-20 mins. Do some breathwork. Stretch 5-10 mins. Journal 5 mins. Plan day 5 mins. Gym for workout, yoga or a walk on the beach 20-90 mins. 15-20 mins for learning/inspiration. Fresh pressed juice, smoothie or fruit for breakfast. By 9 AM I'm ready to start the workday and only then look at my phone.

Actions you choose, no matter how small, will help you move towards your best health in any of the following areas:

Mindset
- You are enough! Write it down where you can see it and say it often.
- Be aware of your self-talk… your brain believes what you tell it.
- 80 percent of success in anything you do or want to accomplish is mindset.
- Be honest with yourself… it's empowering.
- Get clarity around your 'Why' and create a vision that becomes your North Star.
- You CAN do it!

Self-Care
- Support your mental, emotional and spiritual self through feeling compassion, forgiveness and gratitude via meditation and journaling.
- Practice self-love by choosing joy and happiness now, not in the future.

- Overcome fears with courage and live by desire, trust your intuition and eliminate people and things that aren't serving you.
- Be kind and generous to yourself and others.
- Be your own best friend and coach, not a critic.

Physical
- Incorporate physical movement and exercise into your day, even, or maybe especially, if it's just a walk in nature.
- Do some yoga for flexibility, balance, core, hips and strength of mind and body.
- Incorporate breathwork to both calm and energize yourself.
- Buy the best quality food and utilize supplements where you are deficient.
- Hydrate throughout the day.
- Find a way to get 7-8 hours of sleep.

Education & Growth
- Become aware, conscious and knowledgeable about your health concerns.
- Utilize the vast amount of resources and events you can access for free.
- Surround yourself with like-minded people who are living the life you want.
- Celebrate your small and big wins and lead others by your example.

Habits
- Change is hard in the beginning and won't stick if you can't make it a habit. It requires daily persistence.
- Win the morning, win the day! Maybe for you, it's an evening routine, or even better have both!

Brent McCord - Canada
Transformation Specialist - Personal and Business Growth, Health and Wellness. Mindvalley Master Certified Trainer
www.brentmccord.com
in brentmccord
© brentmccord

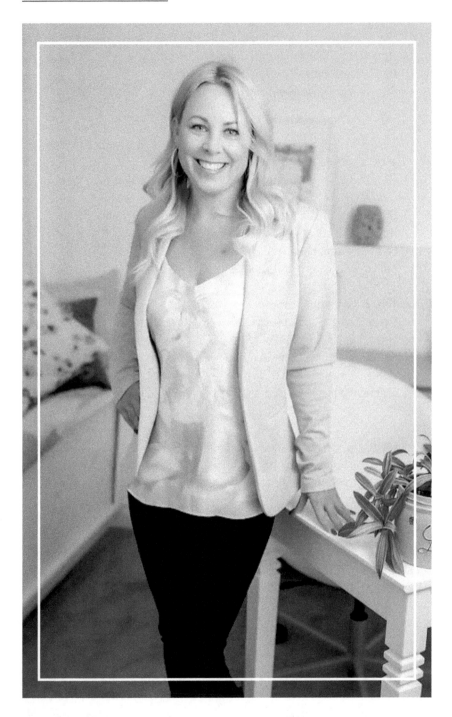

Andrea Harrison

*"You are divine and magical and it is why you
have been chosen for this journey."*

**My desire is to show you the importance of that powerful woman deep
inside you. To make sure you have not replaced your identity with the role
of 'Mama' alone. Let them see you, darling, every part of your soul. There
is no reason to hide or be anyone other than you. I see you, I have been
you… I want more for you. You have got this and I've got you.**

Darling, This is Motherhood

My story begins 19 years ago and I still feel every moment of it in my
entire being. I have never liked hospital rooms. I certainly didn't like being in
an operating room. It wasn't going well and my baby and I almost didn't make
it. I'd been in labor for 46 hours and I wasn't dilating. The monitors went off,
and everyone started rushing. The doctor performed the Cesarean and I began
to hemorrhage. The baby was silent when he was removed and I hadn't even
held him before his Dad was told to take him and quickly leave. I only had a
moment to glance at that tiny little face.

I remember the eerie silence after they were gone. It terrified me. My whole
body was shaking. I didn't know it at the time, but the doctors were trying to
stop the life from draining out of my body. In the chilling silence of the room,
my thoughts were only on the tiny human that I held in my body for nine months
and who had now been whisked away without even a touch.

He hadn't cried when they had pulled him from me. I panicked when he didn't make any noise, thinking that I had failed and it was too late to save him. My doctor assured me that he was fine, and for that brief moment before he was rushed away, I saw the life within him and felt reassured. I had no idea what my body had just been through and, for the first time, I cared for my own life because the importance of keeping my baby safe had taken over every inch of who I was. I had no inclination until that moment that this brand new life would challenge every single part of me for the next 19 years.

When they brought me back to the maternity ward, my family was waiting for me. My son lay quietly in his Nana's arms and the sight of him calmed my fears. The woman who had given *me* life, gently placed my son in my arms. I instantly felt protective, but the feeling of overwhelming love that everyone told me I would feel? That was missing.

Tears were running down my face but I had no emotion that I could name or even recognize to explain them away. I didn't have much life left in me, but what I did have would have fought to the death for this tiny human. This animalistic feeling ran through every fiber of my being.

He started to cry. For the first time, I felt confident he was healthy and would be fine, but the other feeling that came over me, still makes me shudder. I was content to hold this baby for a bit, but I was tired and needed a rest. Logically I understood I was his Mama, but I wondered, where was the person that was supposed to be taking care of him? I always wanted to be a mother and loved holding babies, but when they cry, their Mama usually comforts them. I didn't have the strength.

I started to look around for someone to take over caring for this baby. And, seeing no 'Mama' for him other than myself, panic started to take over my whole being. The stark reality of it hit my heart and mind like a powerful wave. I looked into my son's knowing eyes and realized that *I* was that person for him, his Mama, and he was forever mine to guide and watch over until the day I leave this earth and beyond. But *who* was *I*?

I could hardly catch my breath. I had never seen a prouder man than my partner as he took our son and placed him over his shoulder like he had done it a thousand times before. He was a busy restaurateur and a well-known bachelor who liked to party. I was a server in his restaurant and although he wasn't known for dating staff, we had an evolving connection that started to grow from the very first time we spoke. We had not planned to have a child. We had just started dating and the pregnancy was very unexpected for both of us. We moved in together just months before our son was born. I was barely 26.

After the birth, I was kept in the hospital for five days so my body could heal from the tremendous blood loss I had experienced. My body worked hard to recover the strength that had been drained out of me. My partner went back to work after day two but sent me an atrociously large bouquet of flowers that sat across the room as a stark reminder that we were not going to be the priority.

My mom came to help me each day as I was not allowed out of the hospital yet. On day two, the catheter came out and, trying to walk for the first time after the birth, I realized that I didn't have much strength in my right leg. Standing, I focused my weight onto my left leg, knowing my right was barely holding me up. Getting back into the bed, I had to use my arms to lift my leg up onto the mattress. I knew something was wrong, but I put it out of my mind because I had to take care of my son. This began the pattern of putting my own needs and health last. I had begun to make motherhood my new identity, believing that that was what being a good Mama was all about.

I had so many ideas about what a perfect Mama was. Everyone said it would be love at first sight between parent and child. That from the first moment you held your baby, you would be overwhelmed with a love like no other. My experience did not align with this belief and I thought that there was something innately flawed within me. I had all the feelings of protection; it was my *job* to protect my son. But I didn't *know* this child. How could I? How does one nurture someone as part of them for so long without really knowing them? It would be years later that I would learn to speak the truth to women: your child is not you. You are not your child. You do not yet know each other. It's normal to take time to get to discover and love this new little person.

In those early days, I felt broken. The comfortable and familiar feeling of being a failure hit me harder than it ever had. I had been told I wasn't made for secondary education or a professional career, but being a wife and mother would be something that I could do well, and I was failing at that too.

Motherhood was exhausting. I found myself on my own most of the time with a sweet, tiny, colicky baby with a pediatric sleep disorder. The only time I would get rest was when I would get desperate enough to drive out of town to my parents and my Mom would take a shift for me. There were many tears. The exhaustion and loneliness were all consuming and they almost finished me. And I had not yet found that connection with my son. The stories I was telling myself were unkind and heartbreaking.

Four months later I felt my life change forever, once again. And, I remember that moment with such intense clarity. I can even smell the crisp fall air and hear the leaves crunching under my feet. My leg was starting to regain strength and

I felt the need to get the two of us out of the house. Halfway through our walk, I needed a break. I looked around and spotted the swing set in the local park. I picked up my son out of his stroller and we sat on the swing together. It was so quiet and I felt at peace as we started to swing. My gaze fell on the tiny, cold, pink nose in front of me, and then into his sweet, knowing little eyes. I saw unconditional, trusting, pure, unblocked, unprotected, open and honest love. Tears started streaming down my face. Uncontrollable sobs soon followed. I questioned whether I deserved that kind of unconditional love. I held my son and sobbed until there were no tears left. He quietly snuggled in, continuing to show his adoring love and trust for as long as I needed it.

In that moment, I just *knew*. I knew how much I absolutely fully and completely loved that little soul. I knew I wasn't broken. None of us really are. I just needed some time, maybe longer than others, but in that moment it no longer mattered. It's normal and natural to take time to fall in love with your children. Many people feel like there's something wrong with them when their hearts and minds need some time, but it always comes. It arrives when we're ready to feel it. My moment came when I realized this was a different kind of love, one that would never end.

I made the difficult decision a year later to end my relationship and move home. However, my son's Dad was still an important part of our lives. We would still travel together, spend family time, or all sit down for a meal. We weren't together in the same home but we were still a family. My son and his father had an amazing relationship that was surrounded by talk of pirates and black pearl adventures. The weekends they spent together were so precious for both of them.

I decided to try school again, applied for a student loan and put myself through college. I discovered that I was actually very smart; I had just been bored and restricted by childhood trauma. I went back first for business and graduated with honors despite late nights studying after putting my son to bed. Although I enjoyed the education, I was still making decisions based on how I could best take care of my son. Instead of following my inclination, I felt that a career in business provided good hours and an income to support him. Looking back, I didn't even know if it was a career that I would enjoy. At this point in my journey, my desires didn't matter, my son took precedence.

I worked in business for a few years and realized it was a job that would not bring me joy or purpose. There was a part of me that was starting to emerge, a small window into understanding what would feed my soul. Although this window had opened slightly, it would slam shut when the thoughts of responsibility and judgment would arise. Unfortunately, years ago, a child raised by a single mother was thought to be a risk for negative behaviors and poverty. I decided this would not be my son's story, no matter what it took from me.

Thankfully my inherent purpose was strong and that window started to crack open again. I shifted gears completely and went back to school to study Psychology. I graduated with a 4.0 and loved every moment of it. I soaked up every bit of information I was given and just kept learning more. My son and I did homework together at the kitchen table as I modeled hard work and commitment for him.I started a private practice and knew this was the profession that my life had been preparing me for. Also during this time I married and had another beautiful baby boy.

It was a spring morning in March when my son was eight years old, in grade three. I was cleaning the house when the phone call came. It was one of the worst moments of my life. I heard the words and hit the floor screaming. My son's dad had died that morning from a sudden heart attack; he was gone. The man that I had loved, the man that had given me my son and was my confidant and partner in parenting. But more importantly, my son's best buddy, his co-pirate and captain of all their adventures. We had been with him the day before; he had our son for the night and we had lunch as a family with hugs and smiles as we parted. When the shock wore off and I was able to pick myself off the floor, I straightened up, stuffed down my shattered heart and prepared for the long, heartbreaking road ahead for my boy.

I watched my son walk up the street from the school bus with my heart in my throat. I wondered if his Dad's spirit was walking beside him, lending him strength for what I had to tell him. This was the most important Mama duty that I would ever have. With each step he took towards the house, my heart fractured. I silently committed to giving up every part of myself for the impossible task of protecting him from any other heartache that was to come, and in so doing, the last shred of who *I* was disappeared.

I sat on the floor beside his bed for many nights after making sure he was okay. I would watch him sleep, quietly trying to grieve in the small moments that I could. The realization that it was just me now kept overwhelming my thoughts. I had always had his Dad to help make the important decisions. He was the only other human that would love our son as a parent would. I would now have to figure it out on my own.

Eventually I overcame the grief and took a job at a non-profit agency as a counselor working on the front lines. It was all consuming, but it paid the bills and let me take care of my boys as I had since been separated from my husband.

I worked hard at building a happier and lighter home for us. We would have dance parties in the living room and we were always surrounded by our newest foster or rescue animals. The years flew by as I continued my unhealthy pattern of dedicating my life to meet their every need. At work I focused on giving to others and a lack of unlearned boundaries was encompassing all areas of my life. My health was at serious risk and I needed to make a change.

An opportunity came to train with a brilliant psychologist in trauma based counseling and I decided to take it so I could better support my clients. What I didn't know at the time was the expectation during training would involve resolving my own traumas. This expectation became a lifeline. Two years later, feeling stronger and healthier, I returned to private practice and began supervising other counselors across Canada.

I swear I just blinked and the next thing I knew, I was standing and watching my strong, resilient eldest son walking across the stage in his cap and gown. I didn't expect his graduation to be so difficult for me. In the weeks before, I cried often. I was not really sure why I was struggling so much until the moment when he stood in front of me, grad cap in hand. Towering above me, with his Dad's beautiful eyes giving me that same look that he had given me so many years ago on that park swing. That look that held all the love in the world. He wrapped his arms around me and whispered quietly in my ear, "Thank you. I wouldn't be here right now if it wasn't for you." It was never going to be the same, but it had been perfect.

It was one of the proudest moments I had ever felt. My beautiful son, who changed me in ways that I will forever be grateful for. He was intelligent, strong, kind and prepared for life. Nineteen years ago, at 26 years old, I was holding this precious gift who I was fortunate enough to share with a beautiful man. At the time I hadn't even begun to heal from the pain and heartache of my own childhood trauma.That mixed with the backwards, generational and societal belief that once you become a mother your own story needs to end, made my journey a difficult one. I had no idea who I was now. I had put my entire heart and soul into the last 19 years of being his Mama and that part of my journey and the identity that was attached to it had come to an end.

This does not have to be your story. Let your children see what makes you soar, what fills your heart and puts a smile on your face. These are the experiences they need, connecting to the soul of who you really are. Let them see you cry once in a while; that is real life. Make a promise to yourself to share every emotion a Mama feels. All are magical and amazing. But they can also be raw, heartbreaking, lonely, terrifying and a million other emotions wrapped up in a tiny little blessing, a blessing that will challenge every fiber of your being. And, that is okay, honest and real. It is what being a Mama is… I see you Mamas, and more importantly I want you to see yourself. We are all a beautiful addition to this Motherhood clan, feeling the full scope of emotions in this divine responsibility. You are on this masterful journey of finding you. You have been chosen for this. My heart is with you.

Ignite Action Steps

- **Ask For Help.** This is not the time to show us your extraordinary independence. We know how strong you are Mama, but this was never meant to be just yours to hold alone. Include your partner, family and friends. It takes a village; let yours in. And most importantly... breathe Mamas. This journey is not for the faint of heart, and this, my darling, is why you were chosen.

- **Take Care of Yourself.** We often forget or are unaware of the importance of mental health along with physical health. Take the time to implement self care. See a counselor for support and work on building strong, healthy boundaries.

- **Own it.** Shed societal expectations and forgive yourself for your mistakes. How you do motherhood is up to you; we are all just learning as we go. Motherhood is the hardest journey you will ever take. Don't expect to do it perfectly; no one does.

Andrea Harrison - Canada
Clinical Counselor, MPCC-S
iseeyoumamas@gmail.com
www.iseeyoumamas.com

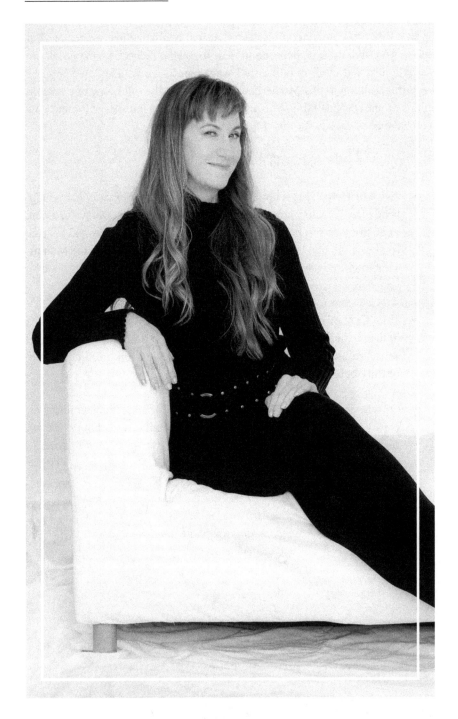

WENDY ALBRECHT

*"Making healthy choices is the key to solving the
illness that others say you just have to live with."*

My intention is that you feel the courage, tenacity and inspiration to discover solutions from what I share. May you find strategies for feeling calm, joy and excellent health.

DOGGEDLY DETERMINED TO MANIFEST MIRACLES

"Just deal with it. It's what happens to women your age."

My gynecologist's words hung in the air. We both sat in silence. I stared at her, stunned. Oh, no no no. I'm NOT accepting that answer. I had gained 30 pounds in a year. I was only 53 years old and had been post-menopausal for five years, so why the sudden weight gain? For decades, I had been dealing with dozens of painful and unpredictable medical issues. I was NOT going to accept one more problem, and certainly not one beyond my control. I didn't yet know how, but I was determined to figure it out.

All my life I'd been told I was too thin. When I was two years old, I started ballet. I was so driven to be the best I could be that sometimes I danced until my toes were raw from blisters. I avoided anything that wasn't considered healthy including cake at birthday parties and carbonated soda. I wanted to be strong enough to dance in toe shoes, which I did for years. Some people harassed me for not celebrating someone's happy event with sugary foods. I didn't care. I listened to my body and only ate healthy foods until full.

I had an incredibly fast metabolism from years of ballet. In high school, I was 5'5" and 105 pounds, which is an average weight for a small-boned dancer. People who weighed more than me would say, "You've got body image issues; your low weight isn't normal; you don't look healthy." Their words felt like a sucker punch to my gut. I worked hard to be healthy and in good shape, but frequent criticism made me feel ashamed, shy and self-conscious. Dancers train like athletes! For my height and my activity level, my body was healthy. Why was it considered normal for professional boxers to make poor food choices to maintain a certain weight? Why was it acceptable for fashion models to starve themselves by drinking hot water with lemon for breakfast to look their skinniest? People would comment on how they struggled to lose weight and had to buy larger sizes of clothing. I couldn't relate to that. I never had to watch what I ate; I didn't gain weight and rarely gave food any conscious thought at all.

During high school, my life changed dramatically. My parents had decided to divorce. To avoid potential bullying in the public school system, my mother somehow found a way for me to attend a private high school. I felt I needed to do well in this new school because I wanted to honor Mom's sacrifices. I was obsessed to earn excellent grades, get into a good college, and find a great job to be considered a mature and responsible adult. School had always come easily for me in elementary school, but I was struggling to keep up in high school. Every night, I would labor for hours doing homework where healthy food and necessary sleep were no longer my priorities.

I was studying so much that I was only getting three hours of sleep most nights. Mornings, exhausted, I would forgo healthy food and eat a breakfast of processed sugary cereal from a box, or toaster pastries. Packaged foods were convenient and quick. I could eat them before dashing off to wait for the bus in frigid subzero Chicago weather, hoping I wouldn't be late for school again. For lunch, I'd eat more foods without much nutrition like pepperoni pizza or macaroni and cheese. I loved cheese and ate a great deal of it! I blindly accepted what I now know to be faulty nutrition advice that dairy foods were a necessary source of protein and calcium.

Over the years, I continued getting insufficient sleep. While attending college part-time, I worked two jobs to help put my future first husband through college. Every day, I was beyond exhausted when I went to bed and when I awoke. My body was starting to break down as a result. I would startle from a horrible sensation of fire ants biting me in random places on my body, but there were no bugs on me. At times, I had an uncontrollable feeling of wanting to jump out of my skin! I struggled to get to sleep. It was maddening. Sleep studies done on me revealed insomnia, sleep apnea and restless legs syndrome. I was prescribed a sleep aid to temporarily help, but over time I couldn't get to sleep without it. I was given another prescription to suppress the restless legs symptoms. Physicians said these conditions couldn't be solved. I believed them and just took these pharmaceuticals for decades.

I saw many types of specialists to attempt to figure out what was wrong with me. Fatigue kept me in bed until I had to drag myself to school and work. Every fiber of my body hurt. It felt like I had been hit by a truck. But the mindset in my community was that you'd have to be dead to not keep your commitments. Not pushing yourself meant you were lazy. I never even heard the term self-care until a few years ago. So, I just pushed on.

Intense pain, exhaustion and concentration issues made it impossible for me to plan my days. I would suddenly get a pain flare from head to toe. How long would this flare last? I'd ask myself to suppress these symptoms even though I wasn't depressed, I agreed to be put on antidepressants so I wasn't labeled a non-compliant patient. I had severe physical and emotional side effects such as attempting suicide three times. I'd wake up every day not knowing what I'd be dealing with mentally or within my body. I was in constant overwhelm and fear.

My symptoms were invisible to others and mainstream medical tests were always negative. Doctor after doctor told me my symptoms were psychosomatic and I needed to change my thinking away from feeling pain. I didn't understand. Why would I create these symptoms? I was not trying to hold onto pain! What was I doing wrong?

Then one doctor said, "It's called fibromyalgia syndrome." I was relieved at first until she said, "There's no cure. All you can do is manage the symptoms." At 33 years old, I finally had a diagnosis — except no solutions to heal me. I knew, without a cure, I had to slog on and keep my full-time job and just work on my MBA part-time. I even switched careers, thinking that might help improve my symptoms.

When I was 36, I joined a company that paid for our lunches and unhealthy packaged snacks. They brought in tasty ethnic cuisine so we could continue to work through lunches. I worked 70-hour weeks for years. I had very little down time between the hour-long driving commute and studying after work to get a certificate in technical writing. Later, when I fractured a bone in my foot at work, test results revealed I had osteopenia (weak bones). I felt like my body was falling apart. And behind it all, I was trying to deal with the constant stress of chronic illnesses, my second husband's alcoholism, and then his death. I also lost my job and had to go on disability due to my diagnosis.

By the time I was 40, my world had been turned upside down. The next decade was a blur of trying to manifest a miracle healing of all my ailments. I saw even more types of physicians and tried every experimental program I happened to encounter.

The year I turned 52, I suddenly gained 30 pounds. I wondered why. In retrospect, I remember I had been eating processed cupcakes and other prepared foods late at night a few times a week. I had continued 'treating' myself to whatever I wanted to eat without regard for my health. Doctors told me the aging process makes the body no longer produce the hormones it once did. I didn't believe them. I knew many people in my age group who did not gain weight.

Around the same time, having sex started feeling like being stabbed in my vagina with a knife! I secretly blamed my partner for not taking more time for foreplay, and myself for not talking about it in a way that he could understand. I kept trying different ways to talk about it that I thought were loving and conscious, but he just kept feeling criticized. It frustrated us both and became one of the many things that ended our relationship. And I still didn't know what to do about the sexual pain or weight gain.

I started asking my friends over 50 about their experience. Most people said, "Oh, I just gave up on having sex. It's too painful." Others told me to take hormones despite the side effects. I was shocked. I was also experiencing vaginal odor and frequent incontinence. I was so embarrassed, since it's such a private and personal area of the body. My doctors agreed with my hormone-using friends: hormones would fix all of it. But I questioned, were all these symptoms really due to my body no longer creating hormones? "What do the women who don't have these symptoms do differently?" I queried. No one talks about any of this! How am I supposed to just accept this as what happens when you get older? Rather than take prescriptions to mask my symptoms, I instead wanted to solve all these issues.

Then one day, I spoke with a friend who had posted on Facebook that she was back to her high school weight. I wanted that too! She was about to start facilitating a program to help people eat healthier where the natural side effect was reduced weight. She was a former mainstream physician and her co-facilitator was a chiropractic neurologist. I signed up for the program called the *WildFit 90 Day Challenge.*

Little did I know how much this decision would change my life.

The WildFit videos and facilitators shared new, verifiable and convincing research on how gluten, dairy, sugar and additives actually cause health issues. We were asked to remove a certain type of food from our diet each week. And each week, I'd muse, "What's left to eat?!" I didn't want to change the way I ate. I liked eating anything I wanted. Then again, I had also gained 30 pounds that way. I promised myself to give the program an honest attempt, so I followed it strictly. The weekly calls were so supportive and the program provided meal ideas that were actually delicious. Over the 90 days of the challenge, I learned to prepare food in a whole new way that nourished my body. Inspired, I got very creative in making my own meals based on the WildFit principles. Friends starting saying things like, "Whenever food is around and Wendy is involved, it's going to be good!"

At this point, the program taught us how to have a dialogue about what was happening on the psychological side of our relationship with food. I was surprised to realize I had been eating what my emotions wanted me to. Allowed to explore that side of me, I actually gained five additional pounds during that phase! I had never weighed that much before and my clothes weren't fitting! I gained great compassion for people who struggle with their weight. We were then asked to go into healthy ketosis (eating in a way so that the body uses stored body fat instead of carbohydrates for energy). With this program's ketosis, we didn't eat gluten, dairy, sugar or additives. No toasted bagels with cream cheese? No desserts? I was NOT happy about these restrictions.

Several times, I felt like quitting the program. One of the facilitators offered Rapid Transformational Therapy (hypnotherapy) which helped me access subconscious fears and self-imposed limiting beliefs. I learned how to manage my thinking and mindset. I saw the information WildFit shared and people experiencing reduced weight, so I decided to stick with the program. The extra weight started to melt away — 20 pounds over eight weeks!

During this program, I also took lab tests. The lab results revealed diagnoses of adrenal fatigue and leaky gut. These findings are significant! Mainstream medicine does NOT recognize these conditions or lab tests as having validity. However, these test results explained my exhaustion that mainstream medicine diagnosed for decades. Further reviewing my medical history, I discovered I had all the factors that contribute to leaky gut. I had been on birth control pills for 12 years. I'd used countless prescription anti-inflammatories for decades. I was on some form of a prescription acid reducer since age 8. I had hundreds of courses of antibiotics without probiotics for urinary tract infections since age 19 after my wisdom teeth were extracted. When I was diagnosed with fibromyalgia, one of my rheumatologists put me on course after course of antibiotics. That caused life-threatening Clostridium difficile colitis with diarrhea and I almost died. Then I discovered something in my research that was incredible: urinary tract infections are a sign of leaky gut, which causes fibromyalgia.

Wait. What?! Something actually causes fibromyalgia? I was so excited! I had been tenaciously researching for 22 years and finally discovered a link. This correlation is still controversial and inconclusive, according to some sources. Regardless, I began working on leveraging this new information to continue to heal myself. I spent hundreds of thousands of dollars from my savings that had been earmarked for my retirement on countless physicians and programs. I was accustomed to making nearly a six-figure income and I desperately wanted to return to work so I could leave disability (that I never wanted to be on in the first place). I wanted to be able to have a better life than the one I was living, which was filled with stress from chronic illness and trying to live within a very low supplemented income.

Interestingly, despite all these illnesses as well as my remaining medical issues, test results revealed that my cell age is only that of a 39-year-old compared to my chronological age of 55. Part of the reason, according to the lab test company, is due to my recent consumption of healthy foods. This finding is contributing to my belief that I'm on the right path to total wellness.

To this day, I choose to eat foods free from gluten, dairy, sugar and additives as much as possible. I now have the ability to acknowledge and handle rare twinges of unhealthy food cravings. And by eating cleanly, I have reduced 15 more pounds and have returned to the weight I was before menopause. I also discovered a gentle, bioavailable hormone through my naturopath so I no longer have painful sex or vaginal odor. The incontinence has been solved with homeopathy. Moreover, thanks to plant medicine from the indigineous people of the Amazon forest, I no longer need prescriptions for pain, reflux disease or bipolar.

If I could reduce my weight and overcome health issues, perhaps you can, too. Eating this way was difficult at first, but it became easier and worth the effort. My wish for you is that you find the inspiration and courage to make changes that will help you become your healthiest self every day and in every way. May you manifest your own miracle.

IGNITE ACTION STEPS

Be your own health advocate. Challenge anyone's opinions as well as your own beliefs. For instance, you can choose to do an elimination diet, or get tested to determine foods that might be negatively impacting your health. Research resources that can rewire your brain and align your mind, body and spirit. Consult a naturopath since they help your self-healing process bring your body into balance.

Do your Daily Delightfuls (self-care activities to help you handle stress).

- Eat organic foods free of gluten, dairy, sugar and additives. Intermittent fasting (not eating between dinner and breakfast) can also impact weight reduction.
- Consistently go to bed at the same time to get the optimum restorative sleep.
- Add activity by walking and doing yoga or stretches.
- Smile often! The feel-good neurotransmitters (dopamine, endorphins, and serotonin) are released when you even just flash a smile. Smiling not only relaxes you, but can also lower your heart rate and blood pressure.
- Meditate to binaural beats (different frequency tones in each ear using headphones). Use alpha waves to foster an alert mind and theta waves to relax before bed.
- Do the rest-and-digest yoga asana. Lay with your back on the floor and your buttocks touching a wall. Rest your heels and straight legs on the wall at a 90-degree angle to the floor. This position can calm your nervous system at any time during the day and before bed.

Create a Happiness Kit. You can easily think of solutions when you have a positive attitude. Include things such as a spray bottle with spring water and an essential oil of lavender for calmness. This scent can be a positive trigger when you need a quick attitude adjustment, as can a journal of your favorite quotes, a list of what you're thankful for, or a list of things that bring you joy.

Wendy Albrecht - United States
Positive Change Catalyst
www.WendyAlbrecht.com
WendyTheDuchess
TranscendentalArtExperiences
DuchessMermaid
AlbrechtWendy

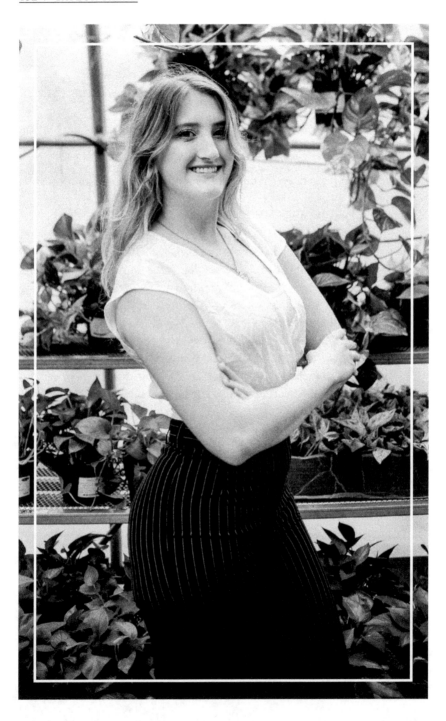

TAYLOR RIBAR

"You are as adaptable as you choose to be."

Through my story about emotional and physical healing, I hope you will feel energized, inspired and comforted on your own journey. Every obstacle is an opportunity for growth, so fight to be more than you ever dreamed, by giving yourself the tools to thrive.

AIN'T NO MOUNTAIN HIGH ENOUGH

A couple years ago, I was sitting in my parked car on the top level of a parking garage, looking out over the city. I had the back seat folded down so I could fit in a set of mesh drawers to hold all my clothes. I had a couple blankets folded to the side and a bag full of snacks in the passenger seat. Despite endless possibilities, I had no idea where to go.

Normally, I had a plan; but that night, I found myself stalling like the engine of my parked car. I thought the hard part was over. If my life was a superhero story, I wouldn't be in this mess because I would have already been bitten by a radioactive spider and on to bigger and better things.

As I aimlessly tapped my thumbs on the steering wheel, I began to relive memory flashes of what the past 10 years had been like. I got a glimpse of who I used to be before all the pain... the carefree, wild-spirited kid who felt so loved by her father... then the moment it all changed, as I helplessly watched my loving, bear-hug giving father be destroyed by cancer. Another moment of helplessness... when I was told that I was going to be living with my mother, diagnosed with Borderline Personality Disorder. A memory of a year later... sitting at the lunch table unable to relate to my peers because my good days were spent tiptoeing into the house without waking my mom so she wouldn't yell or throw things. A flash of embarrassment... having to leave class to talk to a Child Protective Services Officer as things kept getting worse. A moment of relief... when the teacher would let me leave class to go to the bathroom so I could cry or have a panic attack in the privacy of a bathroom stall. A flash of me as a senior in highschool... having bounced around in living situations, never feeling heard, loved or accepted anywhere I tried to go.

I was utterly exhausted.

In that moment, sitting in my car, I had given up trying to be anything more than the shell of the girl I had become. Ten years of stress, trauma and anxiety had manifested into a person who did not believe she was smart, capable, beautiful or able to make a difference in either her life or the lives of others. I had become a mixture of what people told me to be, thought I should be or said I could or could not do. I craved a place that felt like home. I thought my life was going to be very different. I wondered why it had all happened and the reasons I still felt the ache and pain as if it was yesterday. The loss felt heavy in my chest, as if I could not take a full breath. Little did I know, the leftover pain from my past was trying to shine a beacon on the parts of myself that needed healing.

That summer I was at a standstill, in between cities and colleges, waiting on a school acceptance letter before finding an apartment to begin the next phase of my life. Temporarily homeless, every few days, I would drag my bag out of my car and into somewhere new, but with every new place came a new set of expectations of what I should do or who I should be and just never felt like *home*.

With too much time to think and too little freedom to discover who I was, I found myself becoming more and more anxious and spending late nights overthinking everything. My mind felt like the moment in the old Western movies when the stagecoach driver loses the reins on the horses so the carriage just barrels along without direction or control. My anxiety often spiraled out of control.

In this period of my life, I was just trying to survive. I did not know if my mind even had any reins or if I could find them if it did. It was at this time I had a key realization and I knew I needed to take a risk.

If my life were a Western movie, two things could happen. Either I could let the stagecoach horses run reinless, where they would inevitably find a cliff to run off of. Or... I could take the risk I needed to try to get a hold of the reins.

That summer, moving around, I realized I could keep being unhappy and let the direction of my life be dictated by fear, chaos and other people or I could find a way to grasp control of my life and move towards the future I wanted.

The first step was determining what I could change in my present situation. I could not pinpoint the specific ways I needed to heal *emotionally*, so I decided to start healing and growing *physically*. In an attempt to moderate my anxiety, I did some physical activity everyday. I even developed a system where, if I started feeling anxious, I would do 25 jumping jacks or 5 push-ups. Exercise allowed me to forcibly raise my energy to a higher level whenever emotional wounds that I wasn't ready to address started to drag me down. Slowly, with many repetitions, I began to feel better than I had in years.

As the summer was ending, I moved into my first apartment. The bathroom was so small you could barely close the door and fit in it to use it. There was an old musty smell that persisted no matter how many candles I burned. It wasn't fancy, but it was safe; it was consistent and it was mine.

Within weeks, I was lying on my living room floor feeling utterly alone. I felt like I was missing the final piece to the puzzle. I had thought that having a home of my own would fix this unsettled feeling, but lying there, my heart rate started to increase and it became harder to breathe. I quickly grew anxious. The air conditioning machine was wheezing loudly and I focused all my attention on that sound in an attempt to steady my breathing. In and out. In... and out. Slowly, with every breath, the idea blossomed inside me that I was not uncomfortable with my *apartment*, I was uncomfortable with *myself*. Confronted with a floodgate of revelations, I had become Ignited.

Having a safe space was not the *key*, it was a *tool*. It was a piece to the Swiss army knife of my mental health and healing. The safety of my home gave me the confidence to uproot and confront the areas in which I was uncomfortable with myself. Casting aside the person who I had been told I was, I desperately wanted to meet my true self: the person I chose to be. But first, I needed to do the work in order to meet her.

I knew I wanted to begin my healing journey but, I had no idea *if* I could heal. I was worried that in the process of healing I would either break myself even more or discover that I was unfixable. Life is too short to give up fighting for something better, so I decided to fully commit to healing because I was tired of living the alternative. I sacrificed effort, and the parts of myself that no longer supported the person I wanted to be. With the realization that I could live a better alternative, I was ignited into action.

I needed a clear vision of who I wanted to be and trust that I could get there:

the courage to seize opportunities for growth, the endurance to make and stick to a game plan. I was driven to take a step on my path everyday. The next two years were a lot of trial and error. I was reading journals, psychology papers and self help books, and listening to podcasts and anything that had insight into people who had similar experiences. I needed to understand what I was dealing with in order to overcome it by calling on the insight of others.

I had a journal where I would track what I did on good days and bad days and made an effort to implement habits that showed a beneficial pattern. At the end of two years, I finally felt better. I was proud of myself. I was in the best physical shape of my life, cultivating my spirituality with meditation and uprooting the negative beliefs, habits and reactions so I could learn and grow. I began intentionally cultivating positive life and growth around me.

I picked up a new hobby, taking care of plants. It's as if by taking care of plants, I was reminded to also take care of myself. By encouraging them to grow, I was reminded of how I also needed tender encouragement.

Through growth, I found confidence. Things I once thought were unchangeable were transformed through perspective and healing. Healing is a process, the same methods that healed one wound do not heal all. I had to give myself the grace to try and to fail. Because in those two years, I failed a lot more than I succeeded. But I also made more progress than I anticipated. Progress gave me confidence to fearlessly challenge myself to do things I once thought I couldn't do. But I believe that life tests us. Life tests the lessons we think we have learned to show us areas that still need work and healing.

I took that test on the edge of my bathtub. I felt numb. I had just found out I was pregnant. This information jammed my brain for a long time, then reality flooded in — a flood of uncertainty, fear and doubt. Fear of the future and doubt of myself.

Childhood fears of not being capable, along with new worries triggered by memories of my mother, all surfaced in an instant. I sat there on the edge of the bathtub for a long time, caught in between all the negative childhood perceptions and experiences, and the person I had fought so hard to become. There is nothing heavier than the weight of potential resting solely on your shoulders. But no one is more qualified to make that decision than a woman taking stock of her life on the edge of a bathtub. I was lucky; I was free to choose what to put my soul at peace.

There is a reason you don't see pregnant superheroes. Their battles may not be glamorous, but they are glorious. I remember being five months pregnant, a full time college student, trying to take a biology exam. I had to squeeze into a tiny exam desk with a watermelon bump under my shirt only to have to get up to pee three times in the first hour. It was the walking which made me realize that in the midst of studying I had forgotten to eat. Between hormones, physical discomfort and lack of food, the information I had tried so desperately to remember was sand slipping through my fingers. I was largely embarrassed and embarrassingly large.

I thought that was the worst of it, but about two months before I was due to give birth, I developed Symphysis Pubis Dysfunction, which is the medical equivalent of "Something is not working quite right and will probably hurt." After having felt the pain of childbirth, I can say those two months were the worst pain I have ever felt. I could not even turn over in bed without bursting into tears. Once again I felt helpless in my own situation.

I wanted to continue my personal progress and my healing journey, but many of the habits and coping strategies I had learned... no longer worked. I had strived to be independent and self sufficient, and now I could barely get out of bed by myself. I fell into a deep cycle of comparison because I could not do many of the things I wanted to do or what my friends were doing.

I was jealous and bitter and more than anything self conscious. I was hurting and had a really hard time feeling joy for others. But I did not want to be this bitter, jealous person so I wrote a mantra on pieces of paper and stuck them up around my apartment.

"The beauty and greatness of others does not decrease your own."

"The world will always have room for good,
and all good is equal to the world."

"Whatever good you can bring into the world each day is enough."

I learned to appreciate others without comparison to myself, knowing whatever goodness and kindness I could bring into the world each day was enough. It is the act of giving, not how much you give, that showed me my own value... and that which I had to offer the world.

Looking back I realize my pregnancy led me to develop in areas I had previously neglected. Where I had once worked to be independent, I now had to learn to trust in others. I knew that while my external progress of my physical health and living space helped initiate my healing process, the final steps towards healing, comfort and growth were internal.

I continued to grow with meditation, cultivating the plants and caring for the new pets I had brought into my home. I learned new stretches and workouts that could help relieve pain in my body. Regardless of what was going on externally, I learned to fully embrace myself in the moment as the person I am intentionally choosing to be, everyday. My commitment to myself and my personal journey gave me the tools to get through both childbirth and postpartum because for those of you who don't know... having a baby is really hard.

I distinctly remember being 21 in a hospital room. My beautiful daughter was screaming in a little bed next to me. I was wearing a diaper, feeling like my netherregions were a stitched-up experiment of Dr. Frankenstein, and looking like a half-deflated balloon. This was not the hot mom aesthetic I was hoping for.

After a nine-month battle of growing and changing, the scariest question was "What's next?" There were so many aspects of myself I did not recognize. I gained almost 60 pounds during pregnancy and my body felt significantly different to live in. It was the ugliest I had ever felt in my entire life. There were times I would look in the mirror in shock because I no longer recognized my own reflection. And one of the hardest parts was I felt that my individuality was overshadowed by my new role as an 'all you can eat' buffet for one tiny demanding customer.

After working so hard to solidify who I was, cultivate my healthy habits and heal old wounds, I found myself more uncertain than I have ever been. I craved the comfort and familiarity of who I used to be. I desperately wanted my old body, freedom and independence. But this time something was different. I realized I did not want to once again give up the reins to fear. I didn't want to feel like my life was out of control. I had worked through so much. I had come so far.

I called upon the knowledge I gained from my previous challenges to courageously face the many sleepless nights, endless worries and uncertainty that accompanies the first few months as a new mother. Many of the tools and strategies I used to initiate my healing I have been able to modify to continue my journey. But more than that, my journey has given me the confidence that I can adapt and I can heal. Even as life tests you, you can learn, practice and implement habits that will help you achieve your highest aspirations.

The life I have cultivated around me comforts me in times I feel alone. Becoming a mother has inspired me to encourage my daughter to be like the confident, carefree, wild-spirited kid I once was. My challenges have given me opportunities to grow and allowed me to intentionally tailor my life towards a life I only dared to dream.

You can live the life you always wanted as long as you have the courage and determination to live ignited.

IGNITE ACTION STEPS

Four Ways to Initiate Healing and Growth

- **Take care of your mind:** The mind is a muscle that can grow and develop. A healthy mind can initiate and motivate a journey towards your highest ambition. Nourish your mind with knowledge, positivity, mindfulness and meditation, and watch it blossom into an advocate for your most authentic self.

- **Take care of your body**: The more we take care of our body, the more energy and ability it can offer us on our journey to connecting and experiencing the world. Nourish your body with the food it needs and physical activity it craves, and watch your ability to act out your intentions increase.

- **Take care of your environment:** Your external environment can often mirror your internal environment. If you take care to create a space that is a source of innovation, inspiration and energy, your space will in turn take care of you.

- **Take care of life:** Selflessly and mindfully cultivating life around you has the potential to break negative self-absorbed cycles through perspective by encouraging you to live consciously and intentionally.

Taylor Ribar - United States
A loving student of the world
www.intentionallytaylored.com
⊙ Intentionally_Taylored

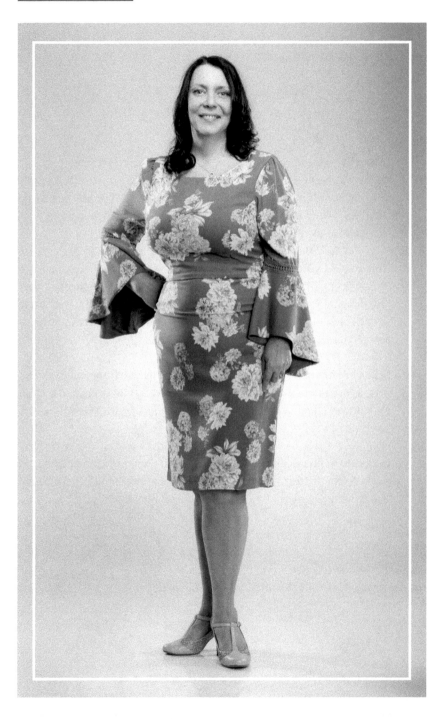

ANN BRIDGES

*"Forget fear and pain; birthing is designed to be
a euphoric journey of joy and love."*

My intention is for you to experience birth as an amazing, transformative process. To create healing and break the negative, fearful and painful spell that we have been innocently told. To forgive the past and liberate the future for women and their partners.To move through other peoples' limiting beliefs, or your own. My wish for you, my dear friend, and the reason for me sharing my journey, is for you to realize that your true nature is more than just your physical body. Within you is your ever-evolving, infinite consciousness. From this vantage point, follow your inner guidance and intuition. You can create a gentle birth for you and your baby.

CASTING A SPELL OVER BIRTH

Once upon a time, there was a powerful spell cast over birthing. It began long, long ago with the burning of witches. The rise of patriarchal ideology overthrew the Goddess energy and She was no longer revered as She once had been. We were in the dark ages with a shift to seeing birthing as a punitive event that women were destined to suffer because of their part in original sin. Mothers were no longer being supported, counseled and cared for by their fellow wise women. As people fell deeper under the spell, women would go to hospital to have their children, even though they weren't sick.

In those days, the risk of contracting something, such as childbed fever, from contaminated medical equipment was high. Dr Ignaz Semmelweis and Florence Nightingale transformed hospitals by working to shift people's perceptions. Until people understood that germs existed, the benefits of good hygiene and sterile equipment in preventing childbed fever were unknown. Consequently, the changes in hygiene practices were very slow. As a result, the story of dying in childbirth became interwoven into our human psyche. Fear was now deeply entrenched and the spell cast more bindingly.

Ever since I can remember, I wanted to be a white witch. Well, a white witch Jedi, if the truth be known. Maybe I read too many stories of wizards and witches, or saw too many movies about Jedis and watched countless episodes of the *Time Lord, Dr. Who* from behind the couch as a little girl! Either way, the dye was cast. Looking back and connecting the dots, it makes sense now... my journey led me to this moment.

Unfortunately, there isn't a clear career path for a white witch Jedi, so I enrolled as a student nurse when I was a mere slip of a girl at 19 years old. Helping others was what witches were all about; they were the healers of the village. I realize now that nursing was the most socially-acceptable option available and palatable to my agnostic family.

I was part of a new way of teaching nursing in England. The approach focused on health, rather than pathology and disease, which is an important distinction and understanding to have in the healing arts.

During my nursing training in England, apart from developing my sense of humor, I was allocated to the obstetrics unit to learn all about birth in hospitals. What an eye opener! It taught me that, when my time came to have a baby, I was going to have to do my homework. I recall one particularly bruised post-operative patient. Her abdomen was black and blue. She had had a Cesarean that was an unusually brutal experience where the surgeon had seemed to be punching her abdominal cavity. No wonder she was in so much pain!

The impact of this patient's experience was not lost on me. It led me to write my final year thesis on the topic of pain and pain management. I was interested in how to avoid it, ways to prevent it and best practices to use when you're experiencing it. I also knew I wanted a very different experience when *my* time came to be a mother. The research was fascinating. I learned, among other things, that fear and anxiety actually *increase* your perception of pain.

Once qualified, I worked in the operating room and thankfully I never saw a Cesarean that was as extreme as the one I had witnessed as a student. I was still motivated to look into what I could do to stack the odds in my favor for having a natural birth. I wasn't overly keen on an epidural. I thought a needle into my spinal space was best avoided unless absolutely necessary. I don't have anything against Cesareans. I know that there can be a very real need for one in a birthing emergency. But it is major abdominal surgery and not without its risks, plus the recovery process is less than ideal for breastfeeding.

During my time as the scrub nurse, what shocked me most was knowing that some women were being operated on at times for the convenience of the obstetrician, sometimes for something as little as a football game on television, rather than for the benefit of the mother.

Induction and Cesarean rates have been steadily rising. Has giving birth become more difficult? Or has the spell cast over birthing impacted our collective misunderstanding of the best way to manage birthing? After all, it is a normal, natural physiological process. The body knows what to do. It isn't broken, doesn't need fixing, nor any unnecessary intervention. *Birth doesn't have to be a huge medical event.* With a deeper understanding of birth and the natural magical world of endorphins, a whole world of pain can be prevented.

When I was pregnant with my first child, Lauren, or the Wiggler Giggler as we nicknamed her, I was keen to find ways to prevent an epidural. I don't mind giving needles, I am just not overly keen on having them! I was *determined* to avoid the major abdominal surgery of a Cesarean section as well. I did my due diligence and found that in Australia, where I lived, a birthing center was my best shot at a minimal interventionist route. It was more difficult at that time to have a homebirth in Australia, and I wanted a water birth, which wasn't practical in a second story flat!

During my pregnancy, I developed gestational diabetes. I was fortunate that this could be managed by being careful with my diet. I didn't require insulin injections. I was very comfortable managing diabetes, as I was by then a community nurse and often involved in the education and management of the condition. With gestational diabetes, it was mandatory to attend the hospital clinic regularly to monitor how I was tracking, and I would see the obstetrician at these visits.

During the last trimester of my pregnancy, I had waited and waited. (I think this is why we are given the name of patient, because patience has to be cultivated in hospital!) I sat in the noisy and bustling waiting room, filled with pregnant women and their young babies. When I finally got to see the obstetrician, he was sitting behind an imposing wooden desk, wearing his bow tie and white coat. He was the quintessential consultant. He peered at me from over his glasses for the briefest of moments and then went back to reading the notes on me. After a few moments spent in silence, he finally came around the desk and perched himself on the corner closest to me. Looking down from his lofty position, he proceeded to paint a picture of the very damaging birthing experience that he expected me to have. He flatly stated, "You have gestational diabetes, which means you will more than likely have a big baby, so you will need an epidural. As the baby is so large, it will probably get stuck and you will then require an emergency Cesarean. So, you might as well give your consent for an elective Cesarean now." He proceeded to hand me the operation consent form in a matter-of-fact way, clearly expecting my compliance.

I was upset! I couldn't believe what I was hearing. My worst nightmare was being shown to me. My hands were clammy. I felt defeated and small. Speechless, I couldn't respond straight away. My brain was scrambled and I struggled to comprehend his horrible forecast.

Eventually, my courage returned. Luckily, I remembered all my experience in the medical world and I wasn't going to let his white coat and bow tie intimidate me! This was *my* baby and *my* birth experience, and I wasn't willing to hand it over to him just like that. I had seen too much. I spoke in a firm, even tone, "Thank you, I appreciate your opinion and I won't be booking in for a Cesarean." And I handed the consent form back.

I know that, in his eyes, he was doing his best for me, yet it seemed such a heavy-handed, narrow-minded approach. He was focused on what could go wrong and caught under the fearful spell of birth.

I then asked him, "Do I still need to see the nurse? My blood sugars are all within the normal range," knowing that I would have a needlessly long wait back in that heaving waiting room. He waved his forefinger and replied indignantly, "You're not a nurse here; you're a patient!" I shuffled sheepishly out, again feeling small.

After my shock wore off, I realized just how upset and livid his comments had made me. I almost had steam coming out of my ears! This experience reinforced for me that women were being misinformed and pushed into unnecessary Cesareans. I wondered how many women he had signed up for surgery with his negative fearful story of birth, let alone how his short-sighted view had impacted all the doctors he had taught over the years.

Soon after this, I watched a documentary, which showed a woman having a Cesarean without any anesthetic! She was using hypnosis. This blew my mind! It occurred to me that if she could use hypnosis for major abdominal surgery, then using it in natural labor would be a walk in the park! I was so inspired!

I found a hypnotherapist who specialized in birth and had several sessions with her to prepare for the special event of birthing my baby. More research showed me that having a doula as a member of the birthing team decreases overall Cesarean rates by 50 percent, the length of labor by 25 percent and requests for an epidural by 60 percent. And, when you have a doula present, the studies show that your need for augmentation of labor goes down 31 percent. Bingo! I hired a doula! Brilliant move! Gwen would be there for me all the way through my birthing. She knew my birthing preferences, provided emotional and physical support, and was an advocate for me.

I was over the due date for my daughter's birth at just over the 40 week mark, although not yet at full term (42 weeks). The medical team was pressuring me to have my labor induced. I had been booked into the birth center, but having an induction would mean going to the labor ward. There, they did a 'strip and stretch' of my cervix, which is as fun as it sounds! The 'strip and stretch' was completely ineffective. They told me if I didn't go into labor over the weekend, they would induce me. The weekend came and went... nothing happened. The team's fears, anxieties and bleak picture about my baby being overdue had me under its spell. I dutifully went to hospital and had prostaglandin gel inserted. A few hours later, while contractions had started, they were still not happy with my progress, so they broke my water. Thankfully, things definitely started to move after that!

I didn't want to stay on the labor ward with its bright lights and cold air-conditioning turned up high, especially while dressed in a thin, open-backed hospital gown. It doesn't offer any comfort! Surrounded by hospital equipment, I wanted to go back to the warmth and more homely surroundings of the birthing center. Luckily, due to my medical background and my determination, I made inquiries and happily discovered that the labor ward was full, yet the birthing center next door wasn't busy. Thank you, Universe!

What a difference I felt as I entered the gentle warmth of my softly-lit birthing center room. I could feel all the tension dropping away from my shoulders as I relaxed on the double bed beside my husband. I could now have the water birth that I had envisaged. My birthing of Lauren went smoothly from there. The midwife commented that Lauren didn't look overdue as she still had a good layer of the protective vernix over her skin.

For a moment, I was frustrated as I realized I could have avoided the induction altogether and would have most likely gone into spontaneous labor if left a few more days! An ultrasound scan would have revealed that everything was safe for my Lauren to stay put until she was ready to be born. Especially as I knew that the likelihood of having a Cesarean increases for women who have had an induction. The euphoria, joy and love I felt from birthing Lauren quickly cleared the frustration.

I learned some valuable lessons along the way and these pearls of wisdom proved extremely beneficial for the birth of my second child, Ben. Despite being over the 'guess' date, his birth was not induced, as an ultrasound showed everything was as it should be. Having gained the wisdom to be able to advocate for myself and for my unborn child was a gift. It became a gift that I wanted to share with others.

Pearls, whether of wisdom or natural, are gained through irritation. The sand that is caught in the oyster irritates and eventually creates the pearl. My own experiences were the irritation I needed to fully understand how to serve the women and their partners that I would go on to educate and support through the birthing journey.

My hard-won pearls of wisdom are these: Women are often being sold short. Birth doesn't have to be something to fear, or experienced as unbearably painful and fraught with danger! When done right, it is a magical and transformative process.

As a result of my insights, I trained as a clinical hypnotherapist, Reiki practitioner and doula. Since qualifying, I have been teaching birthing classes and attending births as a doula ever since. I have published a book called *Gentle Birthing* and am doing my best to help mothers create positive birthing experiences and finally break the spell cast over birth, to bring birth out of fear and pain and back into joy and love.

This is my wish for you. I hope that you have seen through my birthing journey that the birth experience does not have to be filled with fear and pain. Connect with your own innate inner white witch Jedi. You are more powerful than you may realize. Be grateful for the opportunity to give birth and be in awe of the amazing transformation that it brings. You can have a birthing experience that uplifts you and leaves you feeling euphoric, as nature intended.

For those of you reading who are men, your role in the birthing process is essential. I teach men to be an advocate for both the woman and the child by being the strong gatekeeper and solid support. Your presence is vital in creating an ideal atmosphere for the arrival of the baby.

IGNITE ACTION STEPS

Do your research. Find your ideal birth support team who are in alignment with the vision of your birthing experience. Ask your obstetrician about their Cesarean rate. If it's high, you might want to consider an alternative option, going to a birth center or having a midwife at home. Home birth can be amazing and a much more intimate and gentle experience.

Trust your body. It knows exactly what to do and it has a cornucopia of natural endorphins to assist you on your birthing journey. Being relaxed, breathing deeply and remembering that your body knows what it is supposed to do. Understand and trust this. It will dramatically improve your outcome. Remember that fear and anxiety increase your perception of pain.

Surrender yourself over to your birthing body. Let go of the illusion of control. You are so much more than just your physical body. As the French philosopher Pierre Teilhard de Chardonnay realized, you are a spiritual being having a human experience and so is your baby.

A good birth starts your parenting experience off on the right foot.

Ann Bridges - Australia
Founder of Gentle Birthing, Registered nurse,
Energy healer, Clarity coach and facilitator
www.energyflow.com.au
⊙ gentle_birthing

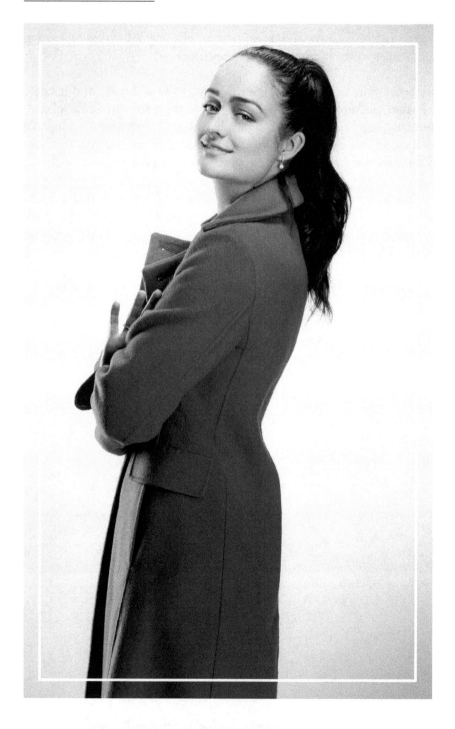

KATELIN GREGG

"Sometimes you have to disconnect to reconnect with yourself —
it takes awareness and drive to want to pilot our own lives."

My intention is to inspire you to manage your time effectively around technology and social media platforms, and to be aware there is a risk of being consumed by them. I wish to encourage you to spend less time on your devices and live in the present moment, connecting with those around you. To also realize that social media can create unrealistic expectations and comparing oneself to others truly robs us from being grateful for ourselves.

CONNECTED-DISCONNECTEDNESS

SPLASH!

My ears pricked and mouth dropped as I realized what had just happened. Peering over the edge of the pool, I watched my iPhone™ sink to the bottom. I had been so engrossed with walking with my head in my phone, I was disengaged from my surroundings, and tripped — throwing it straight into the pool. Fully clothed, I instinctively yet ridiculously jumped in to retrieve and resurrect the device that I relied so heavily on. But it was too late. The phone had spent enough time submerged in the water and was completely dead. Dripping wet with my outfit ruined, my heart sunk... But all I cared about was, "How will I take photos or add to my story on Instagram??"

This happened whilst I was in Thailand, celebrating my graduation after finishing my five year degree. I had been relaxing by the pool every day to 'switch off' but to be honest, I spent more time 'switching on' my phone. Being a millennial, having a constant need to be connected to my friends and family around the world, I was consumed with updating everybody on the *great* holiday I was on and not fully enjoying the rest and recuperation I was seeking.

With 10 days left of the trip, I questioned how I would keep myself entertained and stay in touch with everybody back home. It felt as though a part of me was now missing; I had lost the constant companion I found in my phone. Little did I know, this would be a turning point for me to reconnect with myself and completely enjoy the holiday with little distraction or FOMO (fear of missing out) of what other people were doing.

On day one, I awoke, reached for my phone and felt an immediate sense of disappointment as I realized that it was not there. Usually that would be the first thing I would do. Roll over, yank my phone off the charger and spend the first hour of my morning scrolling through it to fill my mind with what I had missed during my hours of unconsciousness. This would also occur right before I fell asleep at night. It was a routine that had become such a habit — it felt like second nature.

Instinctively I knew this dependence on instant digital gratification couldn't be healthy. I had always been aware of how consumed I was by it, but I never really made a conscious effort to do anything about it.

What's both comforting and disturbing is that I am not alone. A study by cognitive neuroscientist and co-author of *The Distracted Mind*, Adam Gazzaley (MD), found that "8 in 10 smartphone users reach for their phone within 15 minutes of waking up, with 62% grabbing their phone immediately upon opening their eyes." But for those "Between the ages of 18 and 24, those figures skyrocket to 89% and 74% respectively." This use of technology so close to our bed time is troubling because the blue light emitted from our screens disrupts the release of melatonin; our bodies sleep-regulating chemicals, preventing a long deep sleep.

Sadly, I fell squarely into this category. But there's nothing I hate more than fitting a stereotype—and there's nothing I love more than sleeping—so I decided to run an experiment for the rest of the holiday and test my sleeping patterns, keeping my boudoir off limits to cell phones and laptops. I set out to gain an understanding of what sort of effect it would have on my well-being. More importantly, it was a test to see how well I slept through the night.

Not being able to stay in constant touch with my world back home, I decided to fill my time reading personal development books I had ambitiously packed in my suitcase that had not yet been touched on the trip. I spent the next 10 days feeding my mind with knowledge and allowing myself to be fully present in every moment and switched off from the outside world. This redirected focus enabled me to look inward at the person I was and identify the changes that needed to be made. I was about to start a brand new chapter of my life advancing into the workforce. I felt a determination within me to restructure my ways and shift towards a better self.

Going out everyday I felt as though I could really take in and appreciate my surroundings. I began to notice the natural environment and pick up on things that once were missed because of the sheer obsession I had with my device. I started to view everything through my own eyes rather than the lens and screen of my iPhone™ camera.

I started to notice the impact this device-less holiday had on myself and my well-being. I found that I was sleeping through the night without being abruptly disturbed by the pop up notifications or the sound of my alarm. Instead, I woke up feeling energized and ready to seize the day. I no longer required my afternoon nap as I was experiencing my days in full spirit and more connected to the present moment.

I had time to focus on myself and reboot my system. I describe it as a new-found sense of freedom because the pressure of constantly updating my peers on my every movement had been lifted. This might sound a bit far-fetched but for people of my generation, it is a frightening reality.

Returning to Australia, I did not want to sacrifice this newfound liberation through old habits of texting, liking and swiping. Once never imagining life without a phone, I had no desire to replace it. I was ready for another experiment, to see how I could transform my life with a complete cleanse from technology. I was lucky as I was at a point in my life where I was transitioning between university and a new job, so I had no real need to be connected 24/7. I could spend this time focusing on investing time in the most important relationship: with myself.

For the next six weeks, I quit technology and social media. I spent every moment understanding the person I was and working towards the person I wanted to be. For each aspect of my life I set intentions and goals: personal, business, spiritual, health and fitness. I began my morning rewiring my brain through practices of 20 minute guided meditations. This was followed by setting three intentions, big or small, that I would then achieve during the day. My intentions ranged from making someone smile that day to finishing a chapter of my book. I also started writing out in the morning three things that I was grateful for, little things that I usually would not consider, that otherwise might have gone unnoticed.

I made sure to connect with nature by spending time outdoors and fully embracing my surroundings. This was accompanied by at least an hour of fitness and a vegetarian diet. At the end of each day, I dedicated 10-15 minutes to self-reflection, where I would write about every event that occurred that day and evaluate how it made me feel and if there was something I could do better next time. This raised the understanding of myself as I dissected every action and whether or not it was serving my purpose. It was also an exercise to assess whether I had achieved the intentions set out earlier in the day.

I did a complete 180-degree switch from the life I had been previously living as I was ready to raise the bar towards my higher well-being. I could leave the house for the day and not feel accountable to be in contact with anyone but myself. By disconnecting with technology, I completely reconnected with myself.

It's ironic because I likened this new sense of freedom to the feeling I had when I received my very first phone. Let's take a step back to my thirteenth birthday. I had just received a Motorola™ pink flip phone. What joy! That meant I could stay in constant touch with my friends—even after school had finished for the day! I would sit up late in bed for hours having pointless conversations for the sake of the ongoing exchange via text.

However, as I grew up and transitioned my time from texting to social media, this began to have a detriment on my mental health and self-worth. Social media platforms introduced me to the world of instantly sharing moments of my life — however, these moments were always the highlights — creating unrealistic expectations for me to constantly be living my best life. People don't share the challenges they have faced in the day, they usually just post their best moments. As a teenager, I was constantly comparing myself with other people and wondering why I was not like them or why they seemed to have a better life than me.

Theodore Roosevelt famously said, "Comparison is the thief of all joy." This was so true for me — I constantly thought I was not good enough, or skinny enough and judged my sense of self worth down to the number of likes I would receive on a photo.

The detriment took such a toll that it impacted my eating habits during my final exams for my High School Certificate. I stopped eating to become the person that I admired on social media and thought my peers admired too. I would limit myself to one punnet of blueberries and coffee a day, barely fueling my body with enough energy. I was living my life for what other people thought of me and not being true to myself. This pressure I put on myself caused me to lose a lot of weight, yet, I was lucky that I had friends and family to support me and notice something was wrong before it spiraled out of control.

Prior to my experiment of giving up my phone, I had always been aware of how consumed I was by technology but never really made a conscious effort to do anything about it. This became really alarming when Apple™ introduced the Screen Time feature which let you know on average how many hours per day you spend on your phone. *Mine was five hours.*

Five hours a day on average I was staring at a small screen. To put this into perspective, five hours a day, seven days a week works out to be 35 hours a week! That's over one full day directing my attention at a screen and away from the present moment. For many people, 35 hours a week is close to a full-time job! However, this still was not enough to motivate me to direct my attention away from my device — it took a catalyst as big as dropping it into the pool and starving me from it to wake up and realize there was more to life than technology! I look back now and I am glad that my phone was damaged because it was a wake-up call to how disconnected I was from myself.

Having done those experiments and now being aware of this, I am able to take those lessons into my new chapter of educating others of how they can transform their lives also. The period of my life without technology allowed me to be more creative and in the flow. I felt inspired by my surroundings and learned to 'stop and be still' — be at peace with myself and see life through my own positive filter.

Currently, some of my work is dependent on social media — such as my podcast I have developed with my best friend: *'Cosmechix.'* This brings awareness to our peer group in the area of cosmetic procedures, empowering women to have access to all the right information to make educated choices regarding their health. I feel a lot more in control of my usage of technology and all the social media platforms. I am now the 'driver' of my time.

Don't get me wrong, everyone can easily slip back into being totally glued to their phone due to a variety of reasons such as work or social commitments — or just the fact we use these platforms when we communicate within our social groups. The world is such a big place for conversing, communicating and connecting. This gives us so many opportunities to travel the globe, make friends all over the world and live in different countries. This is why social media is such a powerful tool and platform for engaging with family and friends. It's not about giving up social media — it's about adjusting and managing our time so it does not negatively impact our Health and Wellness. By respecting our time and managing ourselves, we are able to pilot our future and achieve the goals we desire. But it takes awareness and drive to want to hang up old habits and dial into our own lives.

It is so easy, particularly among people of the young generation, to become consumed by technology and live through devices. In my eyes, it can be viewed as a bit of a paradox or 'connected disconnectedness.' This is because it gives us the opportunity to be anywhere anytime plugged into with our peers. However, it takes us away from the present moment and distracts us from the people who we are really with. When we become aware of how much time we are directing towards technology and manage it effectively we can fully enjoy the connection we have with the world around us.

I hope what you can learn from my Ignite moments is that you can capture and focus on magical moments without technology. That you can stay connected by reaching out in person as the best connections are face-to-face instead of FaceTime. By switching off from devices you can switch onto a higher purpose. Allowing you to plug-in to the present; connecting you to a world and fully charging you with potential.

IGNITE ACTION STEPS

Dedicate to yourself one hour a day completely technology free where you cannot be disturbed at all. This may be going for a walk in nature or quietly reading a book but the goal is to fully engage in the present moment and allow your mind to be freed of all distractions.

Create a nightly routine for yourself to allow a long deep sleep. I suggest avoiding all screens an hour before bed time and not having any technological devices in your room when you sleep as this prevents yourself from gaining a healthy, deep sleep full of needed melatonin.

Notice *'what shows up.'* Be aware of the time you commit to your mobile device or in front of your computer screen on social media — take time out at the end of the day to notice how many hours you are dedicating to any social media platforms. In your evaluation see how you feel about the management of your time and whether it was appropriate — it's not about giving up social media — it's about adjusting and managing your time effectively.

Check your screen-time usage on your mobile phone and evaluate whether this is realistic. Replace 20 minutes of the time that you would spend on social media with a meditation practice so that you are better directing your time at something that elevates health and well-being.

Katelin Gregg - Australia
Marketing and Sales Account Manager
www.mondeal.com.au
*⊙ Cosmechix_*

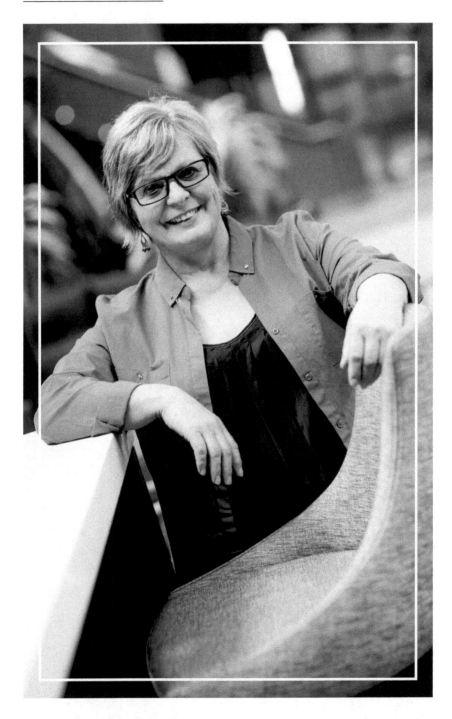

PHYLLIS ROBERTO

"Nothing on the calendar is as important as the people who love you."

We are given warnings, many warnings before our bodies finally break down. We need only pay attention to the whispers, not waiting for the volume to rise. Directly or indirectly, stress is the villain, undermining our ability to resist disease and illness and our ability to heal. Managing stress may be the most important thing we can do to support our health and wellness. I hope that by reading my story you take the opportunity to identify unnecessary stress and be creative in finding ways to manage it so you experience even more joy and happiness in your life.

IT'S ALL IN YOUR HEAD

Catching my reflection in the mirror stopped me in my tracks. The humiliation and rage over being 'dumped' for another, much younger woman, coupled with worrying about money after leaving a soul-sucking but good paying job, glared back at me. My face looked drawn and gray, while my teeth were clenched and jaw set in anger. Deep hollows, darkened flesh and the sharp points of my pupils shook me. Suddenly my muscles tensed as the long suppressed emotions surged up from my feet, consuming my body with an excruciatingly sharp pain at the nape of my neck that raced, ripping across my scalp to explode in the middle of my forehead. I dropped to my knees, clutching my head in my hands, desperate to hold my skull together. I had never felt such pain; not even childbirth compared to this.

A few seconds later, head throbbing in a blinding headache, I slowly crawled up onto my bed. As I lay down, the pain, already unbelievably intense, increased. Carefully, incrementally, I inched my way up to lean back against the pillows. The light from the window unbearable, I attempted to close the blind without moving my head. Even this slight movement had me nauseous and vomiting into the nearby garbage can. Finally in semi-darkness, propped up by pillows and more aware of how to keep my head still and level, I calmed enough to reach for the phone and call my adult children.

Alarmed, they each arrived in a panic. Ready to rescue me, they urged me to see a doctor. I refused. Three days had been my motto for as long as I could remember. If I didn't feel better in three days, I would go to a doctor. This debilitating pain—whatever it was—I decided was not going to defeat me. Everything else in my life was so out of control I was desperate to be in charge of my body.

The only thing that improved over three days was my ability to go from the bed to the bathroom without moving my head. Keeping level and facing forward, I could slide off the side of the bed, stand and walk to the bathroom, and retrace my steps. A sitting position remained the only way to not increase the pain, so I propped up with more pillows, kept the room dark and eliminated all noise. Focused on my physical pain, I could ignore my aching heart and distract myself and others from the humiliation of the break-up and the worry of no income. Like a whipped dog, I crawled into my den to lick my wounds out of the sight of the pitying stares.

For the first time, Thanksgiving was planned without me. I loved decorating with fall leaves and autumn colors, creating the menu to include as much home and local fare as possible. The family gathering was so much fun. The ritual of going around the table and sharing what each person was most grateful for was full of surprises and heartwarming revelations. Love lost, job gone, I could not stay home alone feeling sorry for myself. I would not miss out on this family celebration.

Slowly and carefully I was helped into the front seat of a friend's car and transported into town. Within moments of being settled at the table, I realized I could not tolerate the light or the noise. Barely into my fifties, I felt old, tired, worn out and defeated. Gravely concerned faces followed me as I encouraged them to continue their meal while I retired to the darkened bedroom. Feeling disappointed as I listened to the muted celebration, and starting to really worry, I gave up. I was not getting better. I did not know what was wrong with me and I could not fix this on my own. It was time to ask for help and see a doctor.

Relieved I had finally come to my senses, my daughter Germaine and son Aj were delegated to take me to our local hospital. Although on holiday, Dr. Cameron, the attending physician, was there for evening rounds, so saw me immediately. I told him I was hoping to be given pain relief for this migraine so I could go home and rejoin the festivities.

"Do you have a history of migraines?" he asked.

"No," I replied.

"Then why do you think it is a migraine?"

With no real knowledge, I repeated what I had heard over the years. "I have had a severe headache for three days; I am sensitive to light and sound and feel nauseous if I move suddenly."

He looked at me skeptically. Then I mentioned that the pain increased if I lay down.

Alarmed he stated. "That is not how a migraine presents."

The conversation ended as the doctor went into action. What I thought was a simple fix had suddenly become a medical emergency, potentially a life and death situation. Within minutes I found myself in an ambulance, my 16-year-old son beside me as we headed for the hospital, two hours away. Germaine called the rest of the family, then followed the ambulance to the city.

Propped up in a semi-sitting position, I watched out the back window. I was surprised by my own sense of peace, my willingness to accept whatever was to come. Calmly I watched the taillights of vehicles we met, pass by. As the autumn day darkened into twilight I looked at my son—trying so hard to be brave and strong, his ashen face and wide eyes betraying the depth of his fear.

Reaching out to hold Aj's hand I thought, "None of those things on the calendar—the schedule that seemed so very important a few days ago—matter. Nothing on the calendar is as important as the people who love me."

That was 2006. I call it the year I was so angry my head exploded. After CAT scans, MRIs and various other tests, the actual diagnosis: a cerebral hemorrhage. A vein in the center of my brain, probably defective since birth, had burst, activated by my stressful mental and emotional state. The pressure from the pool of blood created the headache. The vein had sealed itself off so surgery had not been required. After three days of observation, I was sent home to nurse my aching head until the blood was reabsorbed into my body. A severe headache remained for about three months. Three months to think about how I was living my life and make some necessary changes.

By the end of that period, I settled into a new home, a new career and made the decision to be on my own to heal mentally, physically and emotionally.

Massage, meditation and long hot baths, journaling, and long walks in nature became common. Dedicated self-care was my focus… for a while...

By 2009 I was repeating old patterns. Once again frantically trying to fill the bank account to secure my future, I overcommitted to my new career determined to be indispensable. I found myself in a disastrous relationship that completely overtook my life—yet I couldn't explain how I'd gotten into it nor did I know how to get out of it.

I 'awoke' in the University of Alberta Hospital Emergency ward, with no recollection of how I had gotten there. My last memory was the night before at approximately midnight —saying good night to visitors after a relative's birthday celebration. My story now—is what others have told me.

At about 10:00 in the morning, I phoned my daughter Germaine. The conversation started out normally but quickly moved to me being confused and agitated. I was not making sense and started to cry.

Germaine was adamant. "Mom, I am coming to get you. Hang up the phone—I will call you on my cell so I can talk to you on my way there. Make sure you answer the phone."

Worried to the point of panic, Germaine was stopped for speeding as she rushed to my rescue. She found me very upset and disoriented. During the 10 minute drive to town to the hospital, I frantically kept turning to her from the passenger seat, asking, "Look at me – are both sides of my face smiling?"

Somewhere my brain suspected I was having a stroke. Each time she reassured me.

"Both sides are smiling Mom."

In the local hospital I underwent tests for a stroke. My ability to think was not affected. I knew who I was, and was able to recognize and name familiar objects and people. No other neurological problems were observed. My reflexes, balance and coordination were normal. The local doctors had no idea what was happening to me. I was quickly sent by ambulance to the larger hospital two hours away. Germaine, this time with Aj accompanying her, again followed behind.

I was given CAT scans, MRIs, and asked the same questions over and over again: what the date was and events of the last few days, every half hour or so—waiting to verify my memory returning.

When the doctor asked me about current events, Germaine told him I would be more likely to know about Oprah's recent shows than politics. Germaine attempted to trigger my memory by talking of our recent trip to Hawaii. With my memory, I also lost my 'what's appropriate' filter. I had responded, "I went to Hawaii? I don't remember going to Hawaii! That's a fricken waste."

My questions to Germaine and Aj were like a broken record: "Are both sides smiling? Am I still in a relationship? Is that a good thing?" After a couple of hours of answering questions over and over, and the emergency had dissipated, my children decided to lighten the mood by 'teasing' me. My thought process was still somewhat foggy, however—when told I had accepted a marriage proposal I replied very strongly, "I don't fricken think so."

At about 3 PM, I began to remember things like my children's birthdays, then cried uncontrollably when I was unable to recall the date my grandson was born. Gradually more and more of my memory returned. I was told to expect a full recovery within 24 hours—except for the 12-16 hours of the actual event.

I was diagnosed with a TGA (Transient Global Amnesia) typically brought on by: stroke, a head injury (a bump to the head), a shock to the system like jumping into cold water, a traumatic event, overexertion (exercise or overly enthusiastic sex), or psychological and emotional stress. The only possible cause that applied to me was stress.

I had put myself under a strenuous schedule, working weeks on end of 12-hour night shifts, living in a motel beside railroad tracks, gradually getting more and more tired until hours away from the worksite consisted only of making my lunch and sleeping until it was time to go back to work. The trip to Hawaii had been squeezed in between jobs. I was told I had cried that very morning when walking around my yard, distressed at having only been home for two days. All the spring maintenance that needed to be done would have to wait as I was already heading back to work. Physically I was exhausted.

Emotionally my world was in upheaval. The relationship I found myself in was a disaster that I didn't know how to get out of. Trying to be supportive of a teenage girl while distancing myself from her father was proving impossible. I was being bullied and was too embarrassed to ask for help.

In my brain's need for self-preservation, my confused and scattered mind had tuned out and lost the ability to recall recent events. Overwhelmed, my brain was unable to make and hold new memories.

Although these events were different and somewhat unusual, both had a single factor in common: chronic stress. All my self-reflection and life changes had not taught me to manage stress well. There were signs, the whispers I had ignored: unable to sleep, feeling confused and forgetting things. Fearful and emotionally volatile, overeating or not eating at all, avoiding people, keeping secrets and hiding things from loved ones, while disregarding the concern of family and friends. My typical pattern of old was— running, running, running—so busy I was flying too low to pay attention to the obvious red flags that were waving. My old pattern was convincing myself that those warning red flags were actually 'go-ahead' green.

Like muscles that get so used to being tense, they don't know how to relax— chronic, continuous stress had my defense system on full alert ALL the time.

Old issues don't disappear. I still desire to be my 'people-pleasing' self. I don't like conflict or confrontation and still prefer cooperation, working together and win/win situations. However, I have learned that the only person I truly have to please is myself. I do not have to please EVERYONE.

I have learned that security does not come from the outside—jobs come and go and some should go sooner than later. It's important that I like what I do. All those hours I spend at work must be meaningful.

I've been on my own for 10 years. There was a time of adjustment when I felt 'less than' because I had no partner. Gradually, as I became more confident, I grew to love my independence. There are benefits to being solo. I am often invited to meals, outings and as a travel partner; that wouldn't happen if I was a part of a couple. I enjoy my freedom and not having to answer to anyone. I do not necessarily want to live out my days alone. I appreciate the companionship of having a loving partner to share the exciting and the day-to-day experiences in life. I like having options. Now I have the foundation to make wise choices, eliminate stress, do what I like while living and loving on my terms.

I encourage you to create your life, on your own terms. We cannot avoid all the stress we are bombarded with. We can, however, manage and reduce worrying about things we have no control over and replace anxiety with curiosity. We can create rituals and routines that prevent the inconsequential daily stresses from building up into overwhelm. If we live in the present moment and do not worry about the future, or regret and feel guilty of the past, we can reduce most of the unnecessary pressure in our lives. From this place of good health, we are better able to make decisions and handle the inevitable stress of being human. Life will unfold with much more ease.

To hear the whispers and follow the green flags we have to be present and pay attention.

IGNITE ACTION STEPS

Create little habits that you can call on to break the stress cycle. Simple actions like stopping what you are doing to take a few deep breaths, having a big drink of water, posting an inspiring quotation handy to read, smiling at yourself in the mirror, remembering something you are grateful for while FEELING the gratitude, stockpiling a few favorite memories to call on in a second's notice, having a beloved photo close at hand.

These simple things, available to us all, can dramatically increase our quality of life, supporting good health and overall wellness. From this deep sense of peace and wellness we will experience more joy and happiness.

Phyllis Roberto - Canada
Author, Coach, Business Owner
www.prairierosewellness.com
🅕 *PrairieRose*

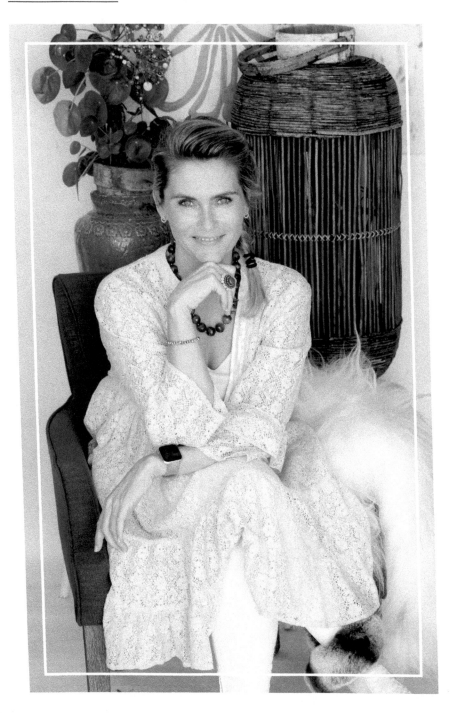

TINA LUNDE

"We live too short... and die too long."

Happiness is not a destination, but a way to travel. My intention by telling my story is to share how 'we live too short and die too long' if we don't make conscious choices and take action. We have the ability to control our health and our lives instead of letting our lives control us.

IT IS IN OUR MISTAKES THAT WE LEARN

Have you ever wondered why something happens to you and you ask, "Why me?" Did you listen to the answer? Most of us don't. We have learned from an early age to shut off when things get tough, and we bring that into adulthood.

In order to understand why you do that, you need to go back and look at your history; not to point fingers but to learn. We are all different. What matters to me and affects me might not matter for you or affect you...This is *my* story.

I began my life being pulled into the world by a pair of forceps. My mom had preeclampsia and delivery was difficult. I emerged from her womb not breathing and blue in my face. The grumpy old midwife acted promptly, turned me upside down and slapped my bum hard. Then, I took my first breath.

My parents were very young. My mom was only 18 and my dad 19 when they realized I was on the way. I was not planned and marriage was not in their cards. But times were tough in Denmark in 1971. Public apartments were impossible to come by unless you were married and marriage, at their age, would require the king's approval. They didn't really want to get married, but their families expected it of them, so they did.

Growing up, I was an only child surrounded by my parents' many friends. When they would come around for parties, they would joke that it was good that I hadn't been just a 'spot on the sheets.' They didn't mean any harm by it, but as a child, it was confusing. I knew my parents loved me, but I also knew that I was not initially wanted nor wished for.

My parents married very young and that brought its own challenges. Some years later, they got divorced and my dad remarried. He started a new family and had three boys, finally getting the life he had planned for. I was not a part of that plan. He left it up to me how often we should see each other, telling me that I could call any time. So what does a young girl who already feels she is a burden do? I didn't call... I waited for him to reach out, which he seldom did. I wondered why didn't he prioritize to see me. Was I really such a burden? I was loved, I am sure of that, but I didn't feel loved by him.

Insecurity grew in me. Why didn't my father want to see me? Why was I afraid of being a burden? Why didn't I think I was good enough the way I was? Why did I think I had to make the perfect decision and seek out all possibilities before making my choice? To this day, I am still curious as to why this was such a big issue and had such an impact in my life. But it did.

Once I started school, I learned I had to toughen up, so I did. I became so tough that I laughed when I was hurting... I no longer knew how to say "Ouch!" when I was hurt. Maybe I was afraid of falling apart if I started to feel anything. I applied this logic to my words, too. I became very sarcastic in my communication and my trust in men was below zero — they were all emotionally unavailable anyway.

It was not until later in life when taking a degree in art therapy, my teacher asked me, "Tina, why are you so angry?"

"Me?" I questioned him. I wasn't angry... or maybe I was...? This made me realize that I was deeply involved in a family theme of resentment and manipulation. I wanted to get out of this negative cycle. I didn't want to hurt anyone. I really needed to work on this, not to please others, but for my own sanity and happiness. My stepfather said many times, "Tina, you are a tough woman! Poor guy who falls into your hands." But I really didn't want to be that tough. It was a face I put on because that was the only way I knew how to survive.

My mom did her best to give me a good upbringing. Believing that public school was not good enough, she spent the little money she had on sending me to a private school. School was never a great success. I was a child who would rather do artsy stuff and play than do my homework. I never felt I belonged there. I often ended up hanging out with the odd or bullied kids. I would try to protect them, be a role model and friend to them. This was a clue. My path had already been given to me then. I just didn't know it.

Since I had come so soon in her young life, my mom never got the education she wished for. At a very early age, I was aware that my existence prevented her from pursuing her dreams. She had sacrificed her plans to bring up a child. I can remember playing on the floor next to her as she worked on homework, trying to finish her diploma. This impacted me deeply and I always knew that I had to make up for my mom's lack of education by making something of myself.

After university, I went to work in the corporate world. It was fine for a while, but I never really jumped out of bed in the morning, nor could I get out of the office fast enough. By the end of the day, I just needed to go home where I didn't have to please anyone. That feeling lasted for years.

At a management meeting one day after I had gone back to work after my second maternity leave, I was looking around the table thinking, "What the hell am I doing here?" Sitting on the couch with my husband later that night, I told him that I would not last for long in that job... and I didn't. In that moment of sharing my unhappiness at work with my husband, I realized that I needed to do something completely different. It was terrifying, thoughts and self doubt went through my mind, but I HAD to make a change. I was so unsatisfied with my life that my mind wouldn't let me get back onto the hamster wheel of monotony.

Ever since I was a child, I felt like I never fit in. And yet I had found my 'people' in the misfits and other oddballs who were not part of the crowd. I felt compelled to help them, to share with them the few small bits of wisdom that I had learned. That feeling, that need to help others, persisted my entire life. Over the years, I had met with coaches and studied with them, always searching to understand and to make positive changes in my life. The Universe was in agreement with this decision and I soon made a complete career shift when I was hired by a Life Coaching company. I was terrified, but at the same time, I felt elated. The pay would be only half of what I had made before as 'European Product Manager' and the title of 'Life Coach' was not nearly as cool sounding. Who was I to give other people advice? What would my family think? What would my *husband* say? He was already tired of supporting me while I was on maternity leave and now I wanted to throw away a perfectly good and well paid career to coach others?

Like all the other career changes I had gone through, again, I was the only one in my family thinking this was a good idea.

Back when expecting my first child, I had investigated how I could ease the load of toxins in my body and my household. I learned how to make my own ecological soap and started using essential oils in an effort to make my home a less toxic place for my child.

By the time I had my second child, I found out I had a severe thyroid disease. I had ignored all the symptoms for more than a year — and I had them all: extreme fatigue, (I had two kids and a new job, so of course I was tired), I lost my hair, (which is also natural right after having kids), I was sore and hurting in all my joints (but I had just picked up running again), I couldn't lose the excess weight after my last child (but everyone struggles with that)... I had an explanation for them all.

It was not until the doctor told me that my thyroid condition would require medication for the rest of my life that I really woke up. WHAT!! I was only 40 and already needing to take medication! It felt like someone had just stunned me with an electrical handgun. There was no way I was going to stay on drugs for the rest of my life. It was simply not an option to me.

I have learned that 98 percent of all illness comes from a prior psychosomatic event inside of us. The good news is that if we find the root cause of the problem, we may be able to solve it and thereby heal. However, I am not going to lie — it is not as easy as it sounds. We are accountable not only for what we *do*, but also for what we *don't do*.

I was already a certified coach and knew I wanted to help people grow, but here I was, more lonely and sad than ever, and sick. I felt like a fraud. How could I be worthy of helping others if I was sad and ill? So I went on a mission to cure myself.

I did more schooling, read book after book and did even *more* schooling.

I did a Masterclass in Meta Health and read a book called *The Secret Language of Your Body.* That was the first major key to my health transformation and healing.

One of the lessons I learned was that my constant aim to please others and my need to make perfect decisions had made me sick. Sick in my thyroid, sick in my constantly over-analyzing mind and sick in my heart.

My generation was one of compliance. We didn't learn to love ourselves; we were raised not to act out. We were taught to have high expectations for ourselves, work hard and not to be selfish. My new learning was that NO ONE would be able to live up to the expectations I had imposed on myself, so how would I be able to?

I realized that as long as I gave the best of my abilities, I have done my best. I found out that 'selfish' is not a bad word. It is necessary to be selfish as long as you don't deliberately hurt anyone on the way. Selfish was a BAADD thing in my childhood, so it took me awhile to understand that 'self care' and 'self love' are necessary to have a happy and fulfilling life.

I realized that I didn't need others love and approval in order to love myself and that I was not a burden when I asked for help. I understood that my parents did the best they possibly could at the time, but that they were only kids and they just copied what they had learned through their own childhood. They raised me the best way they knew.

Looking back at my life, I have had many cases where I struggled with different medical conditions, which I now know I can connect to the psychosomatic emotions that were going on at that time. For instance, in my early twenties I struggled with weak ankles and kept tripping so much I sometimes had to use a cane. Looking at the psychosomatic theme, it meant I lacked direction in my life and was torn between what my heart wished for and what my logical mind wanted. I kept getting sinusitis issues until I left a job where I was being constantly disregarded. I wasn't willing to *face* what was going and truly feel my unhappiness there. Once I left, I haven't had sinusitis since.

Every time some new medical issue pops up now, (and yes, I have not been cured of all illness), I ask myself, "What is it my body is trying to tell me?" Usually, I get the answer. It might not always be what I want to hear, but it is up to me to act. I have the choice.

Changes are not so difficult when they are new and exciting; it is sticking to them that is hard. I'm no different from you; I have not been beamed up by some magical light from space that lets me stick to a plan. I make a conscious choice every single day. I begin my day by tuning into my mental health. If I have hurting limbs or a medical condition, I look it up in order to understand the psychosomatic theme. I then decide on which action to take.

I have learned not to take my health for granted, so in order to stay mentally and physically on track, I have created simple, healthy and easy routines. I put my essential oils where I use them. I have my omega-3 in the fridge so I see them every time I open the door. I have bought a smoothie machine that is simple and cleans up in a few steps. I take care of my hormones (yes, we all have to take good care of our hormones) since they are a major part of the puzzle. I try to reduce stress, which is very difficult for me — as I tend to get involved in way too much. So, I go to bed early and reflect on the day ahead and how to spend my time wisely and in tune with my personal values. I honor these things and they help me stay on track and maintain realistic, healthy routines.

I encourage you to create your own 'realistic' routines. Tune into your health every morning... and this time, listen and accept the answer. Honor and forgive yourself because you deserve it. Your body knows and has all the wisdom... it is up to you to hear it.

I would like to leave you with this note...

My only ambition now (and I invite you to make it yours, too)

Is To Live Long and Die Short.

IGNITE ACTION STEPS

• Make a conscious choice and incorporate good daily routines. I use essential oils and omega-3 to stay healthy. Use what works for you.

• Stop the excuses — don't blame others. Every time you point a finger, three fingers point right back at you. The power lies with you... *claim it.*

• Declutter and detox your mind and your home. Buy only what you need and only if you can afford it.

• Life WILL slap you in the face, but every time you find yourself in a difficult situation, ask yourself, "What should I learn from this?" By asking that question, you help yourself to work through the situation much easier and without blame.

• Read the book *The Secret Language of Your Body* by Inna Segal, or other books that can help point you in the direction of better health.

• Start an Appreciation diary by writing three small things that you are grateful for every day. They should be tiny things: *I appreciate the sun shining today. I appreciate that I had a good night's sleep.* It is proven to work by helping you focus on the positive instead of the negative and becomes the sum of all small things that make you feel happy and content.

• It takes two to manipulate. By that, I mean that you can only be manipulated if you let yourself be manipulated. *Stand Strong!*

- Make a list of things you want to do. When you write it down or say it out loud, your focus will go in that direction. *You deserve it.*

- Accept that life and learning is a journey. We are not supposed to know it all right away. It takes practice, practice and more practice, and that is OK! It is often in the hindsights of our mistakes that we learn the most.

- Get out of your head — you *HAVE* your emotions — you *ARE NOT* your emotions.

- Know your boundaries. If you don't know them, get to know them so you know where to draw the line.

- Laugh at yourself — don't be so self important. You don't have to change, but 'let go' of the stuff that keeps holding you down.

- We learn by modeling; find the right person to model.

- Be present; avoid getting caught up in logistics. Every hour spent on unimportant things is lost; you don't get that hour back… *ever!* Spend your time wisely.

- And finally… remember **YOU** possess the greatest power of all… **The power of choice**.

Tina Lunde - Denmark
Life and Wellness Coach
www.Tinalunde.com
☉ Tina.Lunde

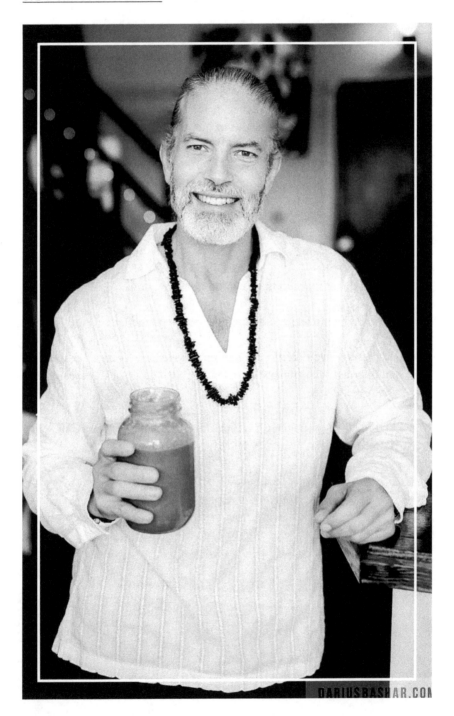

JAMES MCMILLEN

"Your health, Your Life, Your CHOICE."

I want you to be inspired as you explore your health and wellness journey, feeling supported and knowing you're not alone. I want you to see it as a multifaceted experience that needs balance. Your health is your choice always. Sometimes it seems overwhelming so I will remind you with perseverance we can overcome anything we choose. You can become whatever you desire to become; it's in your power. Your vitality and wellness are directly related to the food, thoughts and lifestyle you choose; what are you waiting for? Choose what makes you feel the best!

HEALTHY FROM WITHIN

Many years ago I made a choice, I learned to love myself again so I can be in the best shape of my life, in mind, body and spirit when I turn 50...

In today's world we have experiences and challenges when it comes to life, including our health and wellness. While I may not have known it, my health and wellness journey started the day I was born. But I didn't pay attention to everything I was blessed with till much later in life.

I grew up on a dairy farm. I drank artesian water, had an abundance of fresh air and land, minimal family drama and little stress. My family had a massive vegetable garden and our property was covered in trees and shrubs that produced nuts, seeds and berries. Food we needed was locally sourced and seasonal. I was blessed in this as food is medicine and I had an abundance of everything one could need, consuming nutrient-dense foods with every meal. I learned to grow, preserve, bake and cook everything from the super healthy to tasty cookies and sweets on special occasions.

I was very physically active. Living on a farm there were leisure and physical activities on a daily basis. In the city, we refer to this as functional training; for me it was my life. I played several sports during school and throughout the summer months. In school, I was active in many activities from sports to social clubs. Basketball was my favorite and I played year round. I remember early mornings barely after the sun was up, riding to school with my dad for 6 AM practice. I loved to move. At school I was often in the weight room and when I got my license, I started going to a gym and got serious about being stronger and fit.

There were a lot of other activities and experiences that added to my inner wellness. I was involved with scouting along with my brother and parents. Scouting was another activity that supported my wellbeing; it was social, organized, and we often camped and went hiking in nature. We ate most meals as a family and worked on the farm with my grandparents. Family connection was important and multigenerational.

I traveled often to the United States to see my mom's side of the family, spending time with and learning from different generations as they shared their wisdom. Having family in another country offered different perspectives and experiences that I didn't have staying only at home. We also attended church together as a family within the community. I was in the choir and enjoyed the social times with friends in a different environment outside of school.

In high school, the most impactful challenge to my wellbeing transpired. I was sexually molested by an older male. This planted many seeds in my psyche and created a feeling of unworthiness and deep sorrow within me. I often questioned myself and my decisions, and I would feel depressed and sad. I felt there was no one I could talk to about this and get the help, support and healing that I needed, so I did what I thought was the next best thing: ignore it, box it up and hide it deep within my mind. Little did I know how wrong I was and how those seeds would sprout and grow. This affected my wellbeing in drastic ways as I continued to live my life, not aware of the damage within that I had not worked through or healed from.

I had lots of friends and enjoyed life. I was always out and enjoyed social activities and the consumption of alcohol — sometimes too much. I finished high school and went to college to study business. I was doing what was expected: learning to take over the family business. Looking back, I can now see how some of my activities were offsetting a feeling of 'lack' and meant to boost myself up so I could feel more fulfilled. I was watering those seeds that were planted earlier. My relationships were filtered through these templates and belief systems, creating unhealthy and out of balance romantic partnerships. The seeds were growing within.

After college, my girlfriend and I moved to the big city of Toronto chasing new opportunities. It offered challenges that were much different than country living. Life was much faster paced, louder, polluted and had much brighter lights. Meals consisted of prepared foods and it was hard to find farm fresh produce. My senses started to dull, my night vision diminished, my ability to hear seemed compromised and my well being felt off. I did what I could to combat this by growing my own food and spending time outside, which helped but it wasn't enough. I tired easily. I was eating more convenient foods and diminishing the diversity of food consumption that I had enjoyed at a younger age. Emotionally, physically, and spiritually, I was getting overloaded and had no clue what was happening. I accepted these changes as normal or equated them to some other excuse without looking into the cause. I worked harder and was even more serious at the gym, thinking that was all I needed: more cardio, heavier weights and more food to fuel this obsession with feeling better. This helped, but it also masked the root causes of what was really happening.

I was in a busy city with my partner, dealing with toxic overload from the environment and those emotional seeds buried within. The seeds were the perfect 'Jack-in-a-box' ticking away ready to explode at any moment. I had kept them hidden deep within my mind and I was experiencing a feeling of not being worthy. Being bombarded from the outside and inside, I wasn't being my best self. This turned into habits and beliefs that created personality traits that held me back from shining my light and that compromised my health and wellness every day as I was making the best decisions I could with the knowledge I had. Looking back it seems so obvious now how these templates within me were not for my best self but based out of a feeling of lack and fear. I was addicted to my emotional patterns and was fully stuck in a life that I didn't recognize.

Within this mindset, I was unable to be fully present and conscious in a relationship and communicate properly. This doesn't mean that I was sad. I had created a happy life as best as I knew how and doing what was expected by my partner, parents and society. Many things transpired within that mindset and toxic overload. The box ticked one last time, then exploded. My 14-year relationship ended, my self care suffered, my emotions and mind exploded and my anxiety took over, nothing seemed real.

All I had left were pieces that needed to be mended back together. I moved to a smaller town outside of the city to be closer to a person who was giving me love and support and helping me see who I really was. I had fresher air, was close to the country and fresh produce, and I had my own garden. I loved being outdoors; there it was easy to spend time in nature with less pollution. This was where my inner and outer world would blossom and help me to embrace the real me in full health and vibrant wellness.

My view of health and wellness at the time was a narrow one, but it was a start. Traditionally, the first thing we think about is exercise and diet and little else. I continued to be a dedicated gym person: strength training and cardio were my go to activities. I went every day and consumed food on a very strict schedule, stressing and becoming 'hangry' (angry and hungry combined) every time I was delayed by even a little. (Yes, I was that guy— and oh how I have evolved!)

I embraced a lot of 'bro-science,' (another person's idea or perception of fitness) consuming a lot of protein, carbs and food in general. I was learning more every day and trying different strategies integrating what I had learned. As much as I was starting to eat healthier and stronger, I was still eating a lot as I continued to hide my depression and feelings of unworthiness. I covered up my feelings and hid behind my schedule and obsession with the gym. I was moving farther and farther from who I truly was inside and didn't have a clue as I pushed blindly along this path.

Then one day, I was playing beach volleyball while on vacation in Jamaica. The sun was hot on my skin, my muscles were moving well, and I felt great. But then, my partner's friend mentioned to her that Jim is getting heavy. I, of course, rebutted this with, "I've always been this way; I'm big boned." My ego was taking full control and defending the rounder version of me.

Bro-science had me believing that looking bulky was a good thing. "Let's bulk up before we cut up." There was a problem with this. I didn't really have a plan or the knowledge to get back to a healthy weight. I claimed to be a healthy gym guy, and I did look good to some, but I was at least 50 pounds overweight. I realized that something had to change.

My ego provided me with the passion to become the athlete I wanted to be. I began using a program that had a lot of before and after pictures and stuck with it for three months, along with incorporating my own version of a keto style diet. I went hard at it and my mindset and focus changed totally. I lost over 60 pounds in three months, gained almost 20 pounds of lean muscle and dropped 10% body fat. I felt amazing and on top of the world.

My transformation was very noticeable and my inner turmoil and depression were overshadowed by my newfound physical self. Over the next few months, ever so slowly, a pound at a time crept back until I had gained over 30 pounds. I hadn't realized that although I worked out physically and on my diet, if I wasn't working on the inside dialogue and belief system, it was all for nothing.

Depression, stress, nagging beliefs and unknown factors kept me in a state of lack and feeling that I was undeserving of optimal health and wellness. My food choices were made out of enjoyment and pleasure as opposed to health. I had a daily stop at a local coffee shop for tea and a peanut butter cookie. Several times a week as I waited to pick up my partner in the evening, my go to was an ice cream cone. It was around this time that I experienced chest pain, tightness, joint issues and panic attacks. There were moments at the gym where I was not able to lift because of the pain in my joints and tendons. At home, extreme moments of anxiety left me blacked out on the floor from a panic attack and shortness of breath. I started to feel depressed, as I was being challenged both physically and mentally. I started asking myself, "Who am I and what is happening to James?"

I wanted something more… and different. I knew I needed to express my true self and that things felt off. Again, I associated this with my weight and decided I wanted to learn more and find a sustainable way for me to be healthier, so I completed a nutrition coaching program.

This opened my eyes and my heart to new information and launched me deeper into myself. I became curious about who I was, what I was doing and how I was showing up in the world. I started eating differently, moving and meditating. I immersed myself into wanting to feel more inspired and alive.

In that quest, I attended my first transformation event in Mexico (Awesomeness Fest), and I was on fire! I wanted to experience and explore with like-minded people and there I met many amazing people and had an epic time. The emotional and personal growth exercises I did there helped me get a clearer picture of the life I desired, how I could experience it and how I wanted to contribute to the world. I couldn't wait to implement these ideas when I returned home.

When I got back to Canada, I discovered yoga, thinking this will be good for healing my physical body. I started eating differently and I began to meditate. What I realized was meditation is only part of a yoga practice. Not really about the physical, it was so much deeper. I was learning to move and breathe while remaining relaxed within the practice, not pushing as much and embracing the journey. My ego was calming down as I was getting in tune with my inner *and* outer worlds. My mind and body were at peace in the studio and nourished by the newer choices of food I was consuming. I continued this everyday, fully immersed, almost obsessive, loving it and how I was feeling.

Little did I know these simple changes would be the start of a whole new journey on healing, self expression and self care that would help me create a life of abundance in all areas. I learned that health and wellness is more than dieting and going to the gym. It's about community, self care, connections, sustainable eating, mindset, spiritual practices and belief systems, career choices, money... and many other things. Wellness is a holistic practice with many facets that impact us. In every area of my life, I began asking myself how I felt and where I was within them. I was brutally honest, pushing through my discomfort to find the deeper truths. I was becoming vulnerable and curious from within and was conscious of who I was as a person and how I wanted to evolve.

I surrounded myself with community and relationships that supported and celebrated the choices I make. I rekindled my younger spirit to grow more food for myself, play more and be curious about life. I no longer have inflammation and stiffness in my body and move everyday as part of my daily routine. My diet is 80% raw vegan and I eat consciously as I listen to what my body needs more than what it craves. I have transformed my backyard into a diverse permaculture-based urban food forest. Everything there has a purpose. From feeding myself, the birds, bees and butterflies to providing companion planting and enhanced biodiversity... it all connects. I can work outside for hours in my bare feet, grounding myself with the earth and enjoying the connection I have to the land, which supports my vitality and health in many ways.

I feel it's important to be committed to always improving and evolving as a human being on all levels as you discover a deeper understanding of your overall physical and emotional health. I realized that food is nourishment and whatever I do needs to do that. It now encompasses what I eat, the thoughts I have and the way I move my body. I can now say that I have reached my goal of being in the best shape ever and I continue to fine tune and explore it daily.

Become clear what Health and Wellness means to you. Define it and the goals surrounding it as you find your own 'why.' Your 'why' is powerful; it keeps you focussed and attaches emotion to your journey. I see it as a holistic practice that combines mind, body and spirit. You have the power to choose and I would like to challenge you to make the choice of self care that enhances your health and vitality infinitely. You can have it all: vibrant health, happiness and joy within your life. You got this.

IGNITE ACTION STEPS

- **Start moving more.** Our bodies are designed to move and if you sit for any length of time you can become unhealthy and lazy; the more we move the better we feel. Strength training is beneficial as is walking, dancing and yoga. What do you enjoy?

- **Sleep.** The more consistent we sleep and rest the more our bodies can heal and rejuvenate. At night before bed, limit exposure to "blue" light that is emitted by electronics and LED lights. Go tech free.

- **Meditate.** This has a whole host of benefits. Stress reduction is one of the best benefits as it helps to calm your mind.

- **Eat healthier.** Start small. It takes time and consistency to become unhealthy and it also takes time to become healthy. Socrates said "Let food be thy medicine and medicine be thy food." Consume leafy greens and nutrient dense food as to not be overfed and undernourished. Limit processed foods that are calorie dense and nutrient poor.

- **Drink water.** This is something most people are lacking so make sure you stay hydrated daily. Drinking water first thing as you get up is a great way to start your day.

- **Be Consistent.** All activities we hope to achieve or do better at come with consistent practice. The more we practice at nourishing ourselves the healthier we will be.

James McMillen - Canada
Healer, Speaker, Coach, Mentor, International Best - Selling Author,
Self Care Advocate
www.jamesmcmillen.com
⊙ askjamesmcmillen
❒ James-McMillen-102772161206042

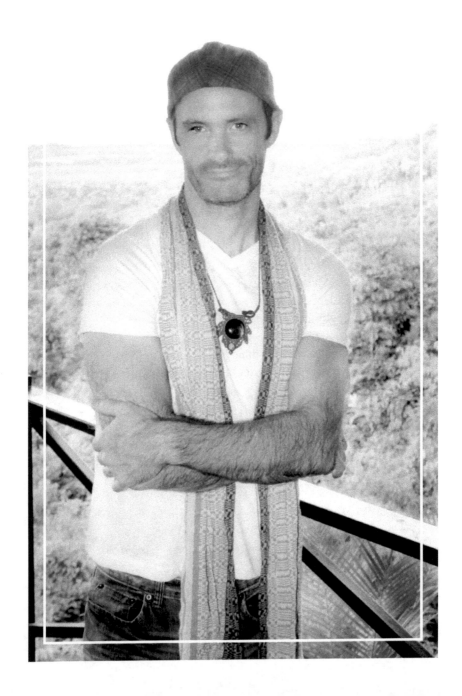

DR. GREGORY DAMATO

"You descended from galactic stardust to this earthly plane to challenge and be challenged. Your soul's deep purpose has been preparing you for this exact moment; the time is now."

Through my words, I wish to deeply imprint the fact that how we eat, think, feel and react are creating real-time, epigenetic changes within our DNA and shaping a new version of ourselves every second of every day. I wish to elevate the vibration of our inner reality to manifest and resonate within the realm of our soul's true healing potential, to lessen the gap between our higher self and our true self to heal beyond the capacity of our own conscious understanding.

INNER COSMIC EVOLUTION

Our 25-year-old hands were interwoven together, deeply in love as we stared into each other's eyes, seat belts tightly fastened with the fervent exhilaration typically reserved for small children on Christmas morning. Our Qantas Boeing 757 from New York touched down in Australia with a small shudder, landing my wife and I halfway across the world at Perth International Airport.

"Welcome to Perth; the weather is fine and 42 degrees," charmed a young, female flight attendant in a sweet accent found only in Oz. Having just been married three weeks prior in Connecticut, us newlyweds had no inkling of how much our new adventure would alter the shape or our latent, indoctrinated realities. Our eyes swelled with wonder with each new sight, sound and sensation as the intense dry heat hit us like a wave while we slowly exited the plane walking down the birth canal of a new consciousness. Collecting our checked bags from our now previous lives, we unknowingly embarked upon the Hero's Journey with only a scarce amount of funds, our soul's contract, an open heart and a mission: become a doctor.

I had made a commitment to myself when I was 15 years old: obtain a bachelors, Masters and doctoral degree in Psychology in order to facilitate my mission on this planet. Now, my wife and I were a team of two united in this co-objective.

Our life-altering journey had truly begun in a hot, strange land of unique accents, driving on the other side of the road, exotically tantalizing food, pristine coral-dotted beaches, new money, shrilling birds, hopping kangaroos, fuzzy koalas and the most breathtaking sunsets. The wonder of it all surpassed any other location on this beautiful planet. We were truly at the furthest point on the Earth from our physical origins in this lifetime in order to create a new reality based on truth, knowledge, trust and infinite love.

After manifesting a tiny, sweet apartment only two minutes walking distance from the beach and a 1986 Toyota Corolla for $200, we had everything we needed to begin our humbling journey. I would spend most of my days researching for my doctoral thesis while my wife would be at her job, supporting us as a restaurant manager on the beach.

About six months into my doctoral program, we were taken by complete surprise as we discovered we were expecting a child. Our excitement was quickly swallowed up by a deep sense of overwhelm and unabating internal questions of how we could possibly juggle a new baby while studying full time and my wife being our only financial support. We remained enthusiastically optimistic that all would work out as we had always expected to have children but much later in the journey. The Universe, of course, always has other plans.

As a young child, I had always wanted to be a doctor to help ease the suffering of those in real need. This boyhood drive emanated from a deep connection with nature, the outdoors, plants and animals and a profound reverence for the changing seasons. This symbiotic connection with nature allowed me to often coalesce with source and dodge the western medicine system as much as possible. I was told around the age of 12 that I needed medication for a disorder known as *Attention deficit disorder* and this medication would help me concentrate more. I summarily laughed at this diagnosis and knew I wanted nothing to do with *that* world. My parents reluctantly went along.

I would tacitly question the reality of many during these young ages and often annoy my school teachers as I never was able to fully pay attention to half truths and misinformation that wouldn't resonate with my soul. This brought about many school meetings and culminated with me being enrolled in Catholic School by my parents in fifth grade. The nuns abhorred my handwriting. One day, I sensed one of the sisters hovering over me as she snatched up my paper while shrilling, "You write like a doctor, but of course you'll never be one!"

"How would she know that I would never be a doctor," I blankly thought. At that young age, I quickly realized that broken hearts are contagious if we allowed them to be.

Around the same time, I was sent to see an ophthalmologist to check my vision. After being prescribed eye glasses, I informed my mom that I had no vision issues and much of this man's income is derived from selling eye glasses so how could he be trusted. I knew my vision was perfect and later on in life had 30/20 vision which meant that what the average person could see at 20 feet I could see at 30 feet.

Upon embarking for Australia, I was put through a barrage of health exams for my student visa. At the age of 25, I thought, "Who had time to think about their health, never mind give serious attention to it?" Once the medical results came back, the nurse informed me of some abnormalities in my heart rhythm as well as elevated blood sugar levels but didn't want to raise any red flags and simply told me to get it checked out when I arrived in Australia.

As a kid, I knew I had allergies, chronic ear infections, eczema, inflammation of the joints, digestive issues and an insatiable appetite but heart and blood sugar issues were certainly new to me. These socialized normal states were ostensibly managed by nothing more than a "let's wait and see" approach.

While my wife was busy nesting inside our small beachside apartment with our new baby on the way, I began seeking answers to many new questions outside of my previous sophomoric reality, such as: What does a pregnant woman need to eat to ensure optimal health for the baby? Should we filter our water, our shower? Should we eat only organic? Is meat a healthy choice? What about circumcision and vitamin K injections? Many more questions that seemed to double by the day continued to flow through me. It quickly struck me how vastly unprepared we were for this unique responsibility of caring for 100 percent of the health of a new, beautiful, tiny human. My all-important, self-involved academic world had been instantly shattered. As I was forced to sweep up the sharp pieces of an obsolete, educational paradigm, these vitally crucial questions were foisted into the forefront and I was forced to rethink everything.

My Ph.D. work took a backseat as I began devouring published research on a myriad of health topics, read book after book and watched countless documentaries. My wife and I had no choice but to apply these new upgrades and significantly alter our lifestyle. We began to implement our research and only ate organic food, eliminated meat, sugar, gluten and slowly weaned out animal proteins altogether, including all dairy. "How did we know if this child wanted to be a vegetarian and who were we to make this decision?" we often pondered.

After this initial research plunge, I continued looking for more and more cogent pieces to the puzzle to get a better sense of the whole picture of what exactly humans need to possess radiant physical, mental, emotional and spiritual health. I knew that each field out there represented a small piece to an overall, unified puzzle. The more pieces I was able to put together, the more whole I found out we could become. This fresh knowledge birthed my love for quantum physics, energetic medicine, neuroscience, Qi Gong, body work and spirituality to help fill in the gaps ostensibly missing in many educational institutions.

My dietary changes began to make an immediate impact as my chronic inner ear infections slowly lessened until they never returned. My severe allergies to grass, pollen and cats dissipated and eventually completely went away while my digestive system was functioning better than ever before. The elucidation that much of my unconsciously accepted, chronic health concerns were being caused and further exacerbated by what I unknowingly put into my mouth, fomented more sparks of personal transformation.

My wife birthed our healthy son in May of 2005 and our world was once again turned upside down in a breathtaking, earth-shattering manner. We were instant converts to the religion of unconditional love and were self-knighted as sole protectors to this fragile, bundle of love.

After two years of our new lifestyle, our frequency began to shift in a big way. We no longer wanted to be in a city and each year moved further and further out 'into the bush.' The more and more saturated we became living amongst the harmonic frequencies of nature, the greater connection and inner evolution enveloped our eager souls. The frequencies of love, harmony, peace and gratitude inherent in the plant-based choices cemented more coherent vibrations into our superconscious with a daily consummation of a full heart and a truly satisfied soul.

We attracted more soul teachers and I began sungazing while eating 100% raw vegan food, coupled with daily meditation on 150 acres of Australian countryside. Sungazing was one of the most intensely powerful techniques I have ever experienced. Each day I would anticipate and calculate the exact window safe for gazing during the magnificent sunsets in Perth. I would stop whatever I was doing, take off my shoes and gaze deeply into the photonic-generator of pure Prana for up to 28 minutes at a time. My childhood psychic connection began to return in a rapid way as I would receive instant downloads from most people I met, like flashes of light of their entire lives in a fraction of a second. The amount of information entering my mind rapidly increased and I no longer needed much physical food as I was *full* on source light. This was the most concentrated form of energy via the circumvention of photosynthesis. I became noticeably less emotionally charged as things and situations that used to trigger a repressed anger in me no longer possessed that power. I became more focused, more still and more harmonious.

My intense research continued as I went deep into quantum physics and applied this knowledge, allowing us to create positive affirmations, visions and goals which manifested nearly as quickly as we whispered them to the Universe. Our growing family's biodynamic veggie garden was booming and the vegetables were often so large that the kids could not even carry them. Their size was attributed to our encoding of each seed with love and intention before planting them. Our outer life began to reflect this newly-coated inner reality and we became beacons of information, wisdom and light for our newly found tribe. I began writing several health articles online to disseminate this important wisdom which it seemed had been greatly suppressed yet was needed now more than ever.

My knowledge and personal soul's journey was deeply tested when my wife fell extremely ill while pregnant with our third child. Having no family to help, we were forced to power through the Dark Night of the Soul on our own as I dug deep into research on herbalism, fasting, gut regeneration, electromagnetic fields (EMFs), grounding, infrared sauna therapy, raw food, juices, probiotics and more. By then, we understood that much of the disease today is a direct result of chemicals and toxins, nutrient deficiencies, negative emotions, EMFs and stress. Now, we needed to put our knowledge to the absolute test.

As a scared young family, for months we fought a daily battle to recoup the health of my wife experiencing severe body pain, insomnia, depression, brain fog, swollen joints, lack of appetite, acute weakness and a host of unexplained symptoms appearing out of nowhere. We refused a purported medical cure and instead addressed deep, latent, *real* causes hidden within the mind, body, emotions and spirit which held the intangible key to true transformation. The typical Western medical approach was symptom management via potent medication for life. We rejected any participation in *that* reality and took full responsibility ourselves to deeply heal this mysterious ailment.

Around seven-months pregnant, as the belly grew rounder my wife grew weaker. Struggling to stand, in constant pain and severe inflammation my wife worried for the life of our unborn daughter more than herself. Still seeking more fundamental missing pieces to our previous puzzle, I continued digging with a deeper penchant and worked around the clock knowing that my wife and daughter's lives hung in this delicate balance. My entire day was dedicated to this crucial mission as I carefully prepared green juices, herbal remedies, probiotics, morning and nightly infrared saunas and a host of other modalities which consumed virtually all of my time. I knew deep down that this *had* to work. Every day was an exhausting struggle as my wife's physical pain consumed me emotionally. We added more and more steps to address bacterial load, heavy metals and a host of other causes that still needed to be addressed. After a month of this extremely rigorous protocol, my wife's symptoms began to subside and her pain slowly decreased while her normal sleep patterns returned and her soul was renewed.

About six weeks later, the last of our fears were assuaged when my wife gave birth to a beautiful baby girl under the midnight stars in a birthing pool with energetically charged rainwater with dimly lit candles in an adorned Native American tipi. We had *all* birthed this baby and knew someday we would tell her the great story of her emergence in the physical realm on this planet under the most extraordinary of circumstances.

My doctorate, in addition to a graduate diploma in science, was completed while learning some of the most pronounced lessons of my life during this time. Throughout this journey, the greatest teaching for me was one of trust. Trust the body. Trust the herbs. Trust nature. Trust the journey. Trust yourself. We have an inborn ability to overcome every health-related obstacle, but we must first release the fear and hold onto our belief in our natural, innate healing ability and the rhythm of our magnificent bodies. Holding on to the understanding that each obstacle is simply a small moment in time designed to inculcate our sense of self-belief, self-love and infinite trust in the journey of life and evolution of the soul.

From this deep journey, I learned that within the holographic, energetic blueprint inside our DNA (known as the frequency of love or the Divine Feminine of 528 Hz) resides our photons (the frequency of wisdom or the Divine Masculine) which recode for every part needed by the body and carry within it the pure code of true healing. From this emergent communion of the masculine and feminine energies via the divine union of love and innate wisdom, we can begin to truly activate the self-heal program from a consummate sense of wholeness. Love creates the answer while knowledge allows for its proper application. The upgrades are here. The choice is ours. The Universe is waiting.

IGNITE ACTION STEPS

Deep cleansing and inner work is a daily process and our ultimate act of self-love and inner evolution as we gratefully and graciously learn to love the beautiful, incomplete, imperfect, perfection we are, knowing there is no time like the present to evolve to a higher version of ourselves. Your body is unconsciously reading from the script written by your mind. Change the story and change your life.

- Listen to your inner thoughts daily as they are the guide for your unique, external reality. Love the ones you resonate with and eliminate the ones you don't.
- Fast at least three days per month to tune your physical vibration back to its inherent resonance of love.
- Smile as you listen to the deep call of nature and shower yourself with her intrinsic frequencies of magic, inner healing, grace and unconditional love.
- Increase your intake of high vibrational plant-based food and herbs as these are the true building blocks of our super-upgraded DNA.
- Using all your senses, walk, smile, feel and act as if you have already achieved your highest level of emotional, physical, spiritual and mental health and fully believe it, everyday.
- Learn to symbiotically balance the mind, body, spirit and emotions to resonate back in line with the coherence of the mind and heart to create a coalescent of cosmic love and inner stillness.
- Your daily thoughts and actions have the potential to be the ultimate acts of self-love.

Dr. Gregory Damato - Costa Rica
Psychologist, Researcher, Speaker, SuperHero Facilitator
www.thesuperheroprogram.com
f thesuperheroprogram
thesuperheroprogram

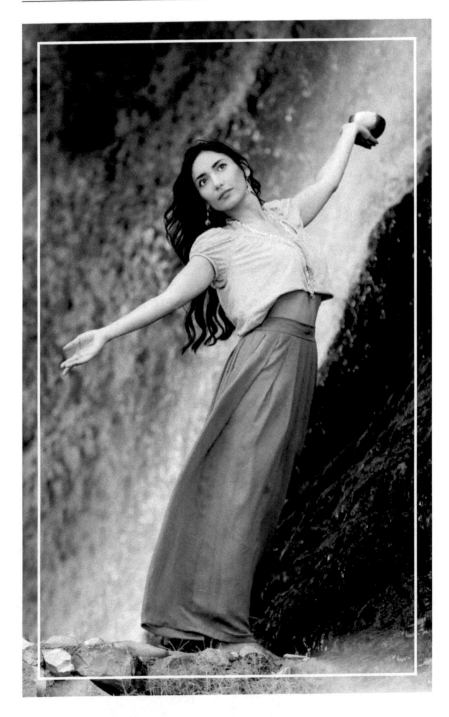

MAYSSAM MOUNIR, M.D.

"Living your best life starts by knowing who you really are."

My hope for you after reading my story is to live the knowledge that you are a Being of infinite potential, of light waves and vibrant energy that are always circulating through your body. Your experiences materialize throughout each and every choice you make at any given moment in time. I wish that you find your way to live a life of peace, light, joy and success. Step up to your magic, actualize your dreams and live up to your full potential!

LIVING LIFE AT ITS BEST!

Born in a family of physicians, with both my parents and many relatives in the profession, I was naturally attracted. As a young child, not a day would pass without me visiting, consulting and writing a prescription to one of my toys in our family clinic. I used my parents' real examination tools and prescription papers in my act.

I worked hard to get into medical school and was excited to learn all about the healing secrets to a long, happy, vibrant life! During the years of long study hours and loads of work required to become a doctor, I kept up a professional, artistic and social life full of the things I loved doing. Aside from my university duties and hospital shifts, I was a professional dancer, a social butterfly, a volunteer, an activist in the community, and even managed to hold down a part time job. Fully charged, full on! I juggled activities that expressed my creativity, upgraded my social and emotional skills and stimulated my intellect, while learning in depth about anatomy, physiology and all the other things simultaneously happening inside our bodies. Everything in my life got me more and more interested in us humans, our magnificent capabilities and the multi-dimensional beings we are.

I would describe my life as nothing less than epic; I was a satisfied super-achiever on many frontiers, walking closer toward my dreams on a daily basis. Yet on the path of becoming the healer I was so keen on being, some health issues started to crop up. I was dealing — mildly and inconsistently — with: acne, irritable bowel syndrome (IBS), lack of sleep, mood swings, body image issues, and many of my relationships didn't seem to work out harmoniously. Looking back, those were stress symptoms in my body, mind and connections with others. It was obvious and clear, but back then I didn't know it.

None of my problems back then qualified as an illness. I was working in a hospital and had consulted doctors and health care specialists on all levels who had assured me not to worry. Logically, since my tests were all normal — even healthy — I shouldn't have given any of those problems a second thought. There was nothing to fix really. My machine was running like a clock... one that wasn't that accurate!

I was able to successfully ignore my symptoms most days and lead a 'normal' life. Other days though, I would flare up and feel discomfort on many levels. Soon, strange things started to happen: my body was feeling heavy, regardless of my 'modeling' shape and light weight. Instead of feeling young and vibrant, I was feeling dull, tired and triggered with acne! I knew life was meant to be joyful and fun but at that point, it felt like a boring struggle and lots of pressure. I lost meaning in what I was doing. Many things dear to my heart transformed into another task to tick off the to-do list. I could not understand why this was happening to me. The feeling that my body and my life were failing me took over and a huge dis-satisfaction took place.

I had to reach into my tool box — our house's medicine cabinet at that time, which for me, was like Ali Baba's cave for medicine solutions — and I tried to find help within the various options available. I thought I needed to energize my life, and you know in pharma, you probably can find a pill for anything! I had magical formulas of vitamins for strength, mood, appetite, concentration, etc., alongside: fiber to soothe my colon and keep me regular, various amino acids, antioxidants, fish oils and other condensed little pills to satisfy my fast, busy lifestyle and new age pharmaceutical needs. I also had an antibacterial solution for my skin and various kinds of creams that came in handy too. It was a 'fix mix' that treated my symptoms without questioning the root cause or reason.

Those solutions worked well on my body. I was more energized and I could cultivate some comfort, but that wasn't the case for my life! I felt like a reactive teenager inside me was the one ruling my life.

One day, as I was waiting for a call back from an agency for an exciting work adventure, my phone rang. The call came in, however, the line was breaking and we couldn't hear each other. This continued back and forth for a while before we lost hope and hung up. I found out later that they had sealed the deal with a competitor after failing to connect with me. Maybe if I hadn't received the call to start with, I wouldn't have given it much attention, but I almost scored an opportunity I really desired. Why, after almost getting in, didn't it actually happen?

This raised many questions and my curiosity extended from how to manage a healthy body into how to manage a fulfilled life. And, I asked myself, is that any different? My research started, and I read an interesting small story: *A man went to the Amazon to hunt game; on the first day, he wasn't successful. On the second day, he wasn't successful either. On the third day, the man had to visit the shaman [the healing man of Amazon] to get his energy worked out and aligned so he could find game. The Amazon is obviously full of game and the truth here is: the man's energy was blocking him from finding what he came for!*

What was that? Energy! What did that mean? I wished I had a clue.

With magical synchronicity, I met an energy master and right away my journey into energy medicine and holistic healing started. I learned that besides the physical body — the one that doctors deal with mechanically by changing its chemistry through drugs or directly through surgery and other interventions — we also have a mental, emotional body that we can affect with our thoughts and feelings. And, we also have an energetic body that is connected to the life force energy. Just like our physical body, our energetical body has organs that have been described throughout time in ancient wisdom traditions. The old Sanskrit word *chakra* is the official name for these energy organs. It translates to 'wheel of energy' and is described as a mini galaxy vortex that is turning, bringing in and transforming the vital life force into physical matter. We have chakras for each and every physical and psychological function in the body. Chakras are the junctions where pure energy materializes into the physical body we know.

The astonishing fact is that *everything* physical actually comes from this energetical space. By keeping this vital energy flowing freely, just like doctoring a wound, healing and evolution are natural results. Why had no one taught us this in med school? Was it just ancient methodologies with no scientific proof? My intellect was skeptical and arguing: you lay down the patient on a nice bed and in a relaxing atmosphere, with calming music on, then you practice healing touch and loving attention... all of that evokes a positive response in the patient's body, just like a placebo.

I have worked with people who suffered from interestingly complicated and stagnant medical cases who have experienced remissions and healing by adding energy sessions to whatever other treatment the patient was following. It blew my mind! This energy thing might actually be working, but how?

My search deepened and was confirmed logically and scientifically. I found answers researching in the Quantum Physics fields like electromagnetics and others. The body is made of systems, that are made of cells, that are made of atoms, which are made of particles, and those particles are made up of energy. In fact, 99.9999999 percent of what we are made of is empty space. The term 'empty' here is not accurate, since the space is only empty from solid physical matter as we know it, but it's full of conscious creative energy with infinite potentiality. Science doesn't understand this conscious energy fully yet, but the work continues to uncover its mystery.

What we know for sure is that every particle in the Universe we know, is a ripple, or excitation, or bundle-of-energy, of the underlying quantum field. Everything in essence is this Energy, materializing into our bodies and every other detail in this magnificent universe. It has been doing so for 13.8 billion years of universal evolution and it continues. Everything that is 'happening' in our lives, inside us and around us is a transformation and materialization of this Conscious Energy.

It's not that 'woo-woo' after all. Everything is emerging from One Source. My hunch was right! Managing life at its best and managing your body at its best are in essence one and the same. To become the best healer I could be, I had to expand my view point and seek different healing modalities. Instead of pursuing a conventional medical specialty, I've decided to advance in holistic medicine. I wanted to understand more about this Energy.

While I was studying about life's vital energy, I learned to meditate. Medical research supported this practice that has promised transformational results: meditation changes our brain structure, balances hormones, regulates blood pressure, modifies the stress response and a long list of other healing benefits, not to forget, its ancient promised transcendental wisdom. I committed to meditate on a daily basis and journaled my impressions, like any scientist would do with any experiment.

Daily meditation practice allowed me a deeper sense of my body. My awareness of myself and the world around me increased. I understood how I was
dealing aggressively with everything! My life became more harmonious and,
gradually, I stopped being so reactive. My sleep improved, I was more rested.
I felt alive and vibrant. I became able to control my moods better, especially
whenever I felt overwhelmed and anxious. I made peace with my skin flora
and with my irritable colon. I let go of unhealthy emotions and any resentment
or dissatisfaction due to unmet expectations. My point of view shifted to one
that's dynamic and fluid instead of static and stagnant. I accepted change in
my life easily and allowed myself to choose differently. Slowly, I was able to
cultivate a better compassionate attitude in my relationship with everything,
first and foremost with myself.

The benefits I got from the practice of meditation made me curious about
the ancient healing knowledge of India. Meditation is part of a bigger body of
knowledge — Yoga — and I wanted to learn what it was and add this healing
modality to my tool box. Yoga (from Sanskrit translates to 'unity') is an ancient
way of living to keep one aligned physically, mentally and emotionally. In
the ancient scriptures, it is described as gradually quieting the mental activity
until it reaches deep stillness and silence. At that point, awareness expands
and connects with the Universal Field of Conscious Vital Energy. There was
that Energy thing again!

According to Yoga, we can access this Energy through everything we do.
Through *Being* and the practice of meditation, through *Feeling* and cultivating
unconditional love and compassion, through *Thinking* as learning about life
on both sides — micro and macro — will lead us back to this Unified Field,
and through *Doing* and choosing actions that transcend one's self to serve the
benefit of the collective. No matter how we choose to access it, it is like flowing
downstream in this Unified Energy Field.

Pranayama (breathing exercises), *asanas* (yoga poses) and *mantras* (sound
vibrations) with all their proven benefits are originally tools to allow humans
the right mental and physical conditions to reach this expanded state of
awareness and maintain it. Whether it's in a meditation session or when
taking a conscious decision, it's all about holding this Energy, and accessing
this expanded state of awareness. Yoga as a lifestyle presents us with simple
instructions and tools of implementation to constantly access the field of
life's vital force and flow with it. I laugh now when I remember filling in
my Yoga certification application. My motives then were all about becoming
stronger, more flexible and able to perform the cool, complex yoga poses. I

never thought that yoga in practice goes even deeper than someone's putting their leg above their head!

In ancient India, doctors used to get paid most when none of the villagers got sick. For each person who became sick throughout the year, the doctor's salary was less! Yoga studies led me into Ayurveda. Ayurveda: "Science of Life" (Ayur = Life, Veda = Knowledge). Ayurveda as a healing system focuses on enhancing health and preventing disease. Health is defined as a balance between body, mind, spirit, social and environmental well-being. Like all holistic health systems, Ayurveda more than 6000 years ago emphasized the unshakable connections between the body, mind, and spirit... long before modern medicine proved the mind-body connection. That connectedness extends far beyond the individual, reaching into the universal.

Ayurveda offers a body of wisdom designed to help people stay vibrant and healthy while *realizing their highest human potential.* It talks about longevity, well-being, manifesting your dreams and accessing a state of perfect health. It gives us detailed and practical guidance to enhance connectedness to the Vital Life Force. We are all made of the same energy. The elements we see in nature are connected to the elements of our body. Each individual has a unique mix of qualities and characteristics that gives their recipe originality and exclusiveness. Ayurveda is all about studying and understanding this unique mixture. This offers the tool kit to stay balanced while navigating this beautiful dynamic life. It is personalized medicine in action, long before personalized medicine became a trend!

Linking simple daily choices to well-being completes the circle for healthy results. What you eat becomes your body; what you think and feel creates your life. This ancient wisdom of healing treats humans with depth and considers their multidimensional nature. It gave me back my power and held me responsible for my choices. It taught me how to design a healthy and balanced lifestyle, and how to course correct every time I need to. It's a system that considers my inability to live life on purpose and achieve my dreams with playfulness and ease to be a 'dis-ease'.

As I observe our world today, I find the majority of our health challenges directly linked to stress and overload effects, bad choices and habits or the spread of toxicity in the food chain and our water resources. We breathe out what the trees breathe in, and we breathe in what the trees breathe out. We are one and connected with the environment around us. Just like the cells of our bodies who work together in harmony for the benefit of the whole body, humans have to work together for the benefit of the ecosystem—our extended body.

We know that the climate is changing, polar caps are melting and toxicity in the food chain and our water resources is increasing. We are aware of pollution, injustice and poverty around the world, yet not enough of us have come together to stop it and heal it. More than ever, we are in need of sustainable holistic solutions of health and wellbeing not just for our inflamed bodies, but also for our overheated planet. We have the intelligence and we have the tools; it's time we focus our priorities.

Today, I'm joyfully living and sharing the wisdom and knowledge of healing and sustainability. I'm grateful that my path as a healer has shifted and changed. I find deep satisfaction helping people live happier and healthier. When you are empowered with the right tools and techniques, you enhance your life on all levels. Success, health, balance and evolution are natural effects of discovering your true Self and your unity with the Energy of the Universe. Connect with the real you, by tapping into this Energy through mindfulness, intentions and co-creating with the Universe.

IGNITE ACTION STEPS

Spend time connecting with the field of pure potentiality, in meditation, in nature, and through cultivating mindfulness, unity and presence. Study yourself — learn about your physical and psychological qualities. Design a healthy lifestyle that supports you and the planet. Create solutions to restore, rejuvenate and heal. Eat fresh, local, seasonal and what suits your body type. Recycle, minimize waste and be environmentally conscious. Above all, slow down. Trust. Receive. Think about the beauty in everything around you and be happy.

Mayssam Mounir - Lebanon
Medical Doctor, Ayurvedic LifeStyle Expert,
Yoga & Meditation Instructor, Energy Master Healer
www.doctormiso.com

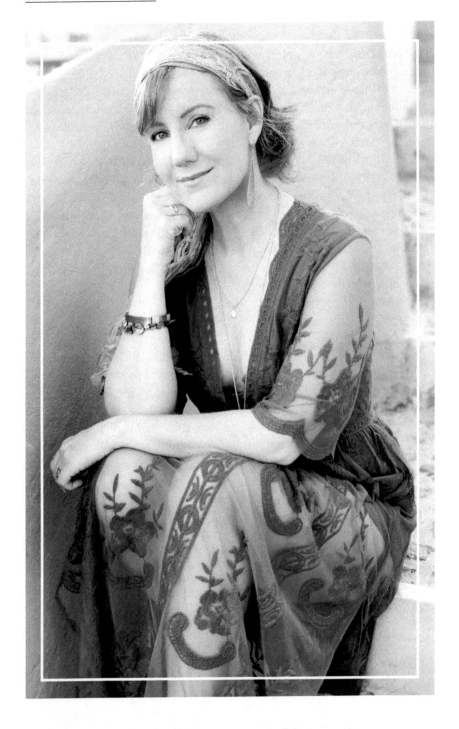

MYSTÈRE POÈME

"Listen to your gut and embrace your inner knowing."

My hope is that you will gain the courage to trust and follow your instincts and become your own advocate. Advocate for your rights, your health, and your life because no one should be silenced or made to feel invisible.

DEADLY SILENCE

Autumn-colored leaves littered the sidewalk and cars rushed by as I stepped into a crosswalk in industrial Atlanta. Seconds later, I was struck by a two-ton vehicle and thrown six feet into the air. A white-haired man driving a white car had been busy looking left while trying to turn right, and he crashed into me. I am lucky to be alive.

Eighteen months after that day, I had not recovered. Once an active dancer, runner, and triathlete, I was now bed-ridden and had lost much of the mobility in my neck, back and left leg. Sharp, shooting pain accompanied my every waking and sleeping hour. If I accomplished the task of showering during the day, it was a major victory. If I showered *and* changed out of my pajamas, it was cause for celebration. I barely counted myself among the living. I was simply surviving from one sunrise to sunset, in agonizing pain.

The physical pain was matched by the emotional pain of having to shut down my creative work as a photographer. I was committed to raising the self-esteem of teen girls through photography, film, and media education. The year before being hit, I had started my company and it was gaining international attention and accolades in the photography world. I was booked to speak at a conference to a live audience of over 3500 attendees about the impact of my work, but could barely keep a clear thought in my head, much less manage the panic that arose any time I had to leave home.

The only time I left the house was for medical appointments, averaging three to four each week. From the general practitioner, to the gastroenterologist, to pain management, they kept sending me to more and more specialists. The message was always the same: this is your new life, accept it, be glad you are alive, and simply take the medication we give you. It seemed like they wanted me to spend the rest of my days sleepwalking through life, like a zombie, unable to function in normal society any longer.

While I pushed back on some of the heavier medications, I needed something to deal with the excruciating levels of chronic pain. The stronger medications led to severe abdominal cramps and tore up my stomach lining. My abdomen always hurt, so they started me on new medication to manage the side-effects. At one point, I pulled out all my prescription bottles and lined them up on the bathroom counter. I counted twelve. Blue, red, white, round, square, you name it, I had it at my fingertips. It shocked me how easily someone in this kind of situation could start dealing prescription drugs to other people suffering from chronic pain or looking for a way to stay numb. And I won't deny that there was a constant thought at the back of my mind that I could so easily end all my pain forever.

I realized how toxic and dangerous that type of over-medicating could be, and how easily it could lead to an addiction or overdose, accidental or intentional. If I could see it, why didn't the doctors? Or the system designed to care for us?

One night, the pain levels ignited even further. I was holding my stomach and writhing in pain on the bed. I sobbed, tears soaking my pillow. It felt as if my insides were tearing themselves apart. My family rushed me to the emergency room where they did a CT scan of my abdomen, looking for something like appendicitis. They didn't find anything wrong with my appendix or any other reason for the sharp increase in pain. More questions with no answers. Predictably, they gave me two more prescriptions and a shot to ease the pain.

A few weeks later, I checked my records online and discovered the CT scan report from that night. I didn't understand much of what the report said as it went through various organs describing shape and size. Somewhere near the bottom, there was a section titled "Findings." Buried in a list, I read the words "intimal flap of the *abdominal* aorta."

I read it. Then read it again.

Having a flap in your aorta did not sound good to me, especially not in your abdomen. I was sure there was an explanation, so I emailed my doctor. I told her that this didn't sound normal even though the lab tech wrote at the bottom of the report that there was nothing to be concerned about.

While waiting for her response, I did my own research online about an "abdominal aorta intimal flap." In my research, I kept running into the term "aortic dissection." There I was, in chronic pain, confused and scared, staring at the computer screen and thinking, dissection of your aorta sounds even worse than 'intimal flap.' I know we dissect frogs and I don't want someone dissecting my aorta. This does not seem good and it certainly doesn't seem 'normal.'

Questions rushed in from all sides. Why did I have this? How did I get this? Was it new? Or maybe a birth defect? I read every article I could find and, again and again, I kept reading about this being a condition found in males over the age of sixty. It's primarily caused by deterioration of the flexibility of the aorta brought on by age and lifestyle. Every single article said the same thing. The problem was, I didn't fit the profile. I am a woman and nowhere near my sixties.

I didn't know the origin, but I knew that I needed to find out. And *soon*. I searched more and found that this kind of injury can also come from trauma, taking a blow, or an intense impact. In all likelihood, it was a result of the impact of the car or the impact of landing on concrete from six feet in the air. Every article I read was a cautionary tale. If I took another blow to the place, that was now weakened, it could be deadly.

Deadly. I was trying not to let anxiety get the best of me and held myself back from frantically calling my doctor every hour until she replied. Instead, I remained silent. I held my tongue. I was being complicit and compliant in not getting answers.

Looking back now, I question myself. Why did I remain silent? Why didn't I speak up? Why did I dismiss my anxiety? And then I remember the previous eighteen months of being told to sit down, be quiet and listen to the doctor. The doctors, specialists and experts who told me that it would be okay; that I had to wait. It was a male-dominated environment and I had been conditioned to believe that the ones with the white coat and letters behind their names were the ones who knew, even more than me, about my own body. And, I had a very real fear of having some type of note in my file about being a hysterical hypochondriac woman who makes things up for attention. Trusting the deeply ingrained belief that they knew my body better than I did, I followed orders. At that point, I hadn't considered or even been introduced to the concept of my own body wisdom.

It was a week before I got an email response from my doctor with a very nonchalant, "Everything is normal, nothing to worry about." My concerns were being dismissed by the experts. I didn't want to be perceived as a nag or get labeled as difficult, but I couldn't let it go. Not this time.

There were news stories and media reports about hospitals and the medical world making minor and major mistakes every day. "Was this a mistake too?" I wondered. "Does the lab tech know for sure? Are they even familiar with this type of thing? Did a doctor actually look at the report? Or better yet, a specialist? Can I get a second opinion? Who would I even see about an abdominal aorta intimal flap?"

I refrained from overwhelming the doctor with all of my frantic questions and just asked if she could send the report back for a second review, or for a referral to whoever would handle my case. I had no idea who was responsible for all things aorta. My sense of urgency was not mirrored by my doctor. Eighteen months had already passed since the accident, yet it took another two months of emails and phone calls to finally convince her to at least send it to a vascular surgeon for review. Less than 48 hours later, an email showed up in my inbox, "Vascular surgeon wants to see you." No details. No specifics. But somehow, the highly-in-demand specialist, head of his department, was available the very next day.

After two months of fighting for my rights, all I could think was that either she got so annoyed that she passed me off and asked him to meet with me to get me off her back; or, I was right - there was something seriously wrong. I assumed it was the former, but at least afterward I'd feel satisfied that the appropriate expert looked at my report and looked me in the eye to tell me that all was well.

The specialist's office was yet another office in the hospital that had now become all-too-familiar. I showed up for the appointment, thinking, "It's going to be like everything else, no big deal, this is fine." Everyone had been assuring me all was fine, so to me this was just part of the process to get answers.

The specialist called me in — *on time* — and pulled up my CT scan. I watched him search through the slices of my insides in full 3D animation. Within a minute, he'd pulled up a section of my aorta to show me what he was talking about. It looked like a pie chart where someone had cut a slice of pie. "It shouldn't look like that," he said. Then he pulled up an image of the non-dissected part of the aorta, a full circle, a full pie, no pieces cut out. "That slice," he said, pointing to the screen, "is the flap."

My vision got blurry. I couldn't comprehend what I was seeing.

While I was trying to regain my focus, I heard, "This is serious, you're lucky to be alive, 70% of cases die immediately on the spot." He explained that there are three layers of the aorta. It was fortunate that it was the intimal (inside) layer and that the dissection was below my organs because if I did take a blow to that area, it could be fatal. I was only hearing a few of the words he said, "organs, blow, fatal." My breath caught in my throat, suddenly afraid that if I took too deep a breath, something would happen.

He strongly cautioned me that any activity that could result in a fall was unsafe and basically forbidden. Bike riding, triathlons, bungee jumping, Tae Kwon Do... all those things were no longer options... for the rest of my life.

If the dissection had been discovered at the time of the accident, they would have rushed me to surgery to put in a stent that would have to be surgically removed and replaced every ten years... for the rest of my life. As it was, we would need to monitor it every six months for the next two years with CT scans, MRI and ultrasound, and if it remained stable, then only annually... for the rest of my life.

The words kept repeating, like a broken record. *For the rest of my life.*

His words were not registering anymore. I felt like Charlie Brown listening to his teacher saying "womp, womp, womp." I couldn't believe I was right. I couldn't believe I had this life-threatening injury. That I had almost died on the spot. That I had almost left my young children without a mother. That I had been walking around with this serious injury for eighteen months undetected, but I had to be the one to look at the report and speak up and say something looks off. And then I had to be the one to fight for months to even get in to see the specialist about this thing that is life threatening and needs to be closely monitored for the rest of my life. All while dealing with the chronic agony of physical pain and emotional loss of my business and all physical activity. It wasn't right. Something was seriously broken at so many levels of the medical system. I had seen inside the system and what I saw terrified me.

It was that moment that later made me realize I could no longer comply with the way the system expected me to operate within their walls, invisible and silent. This was my life and it was time for me to step into my own power and use my voice. I followed all the rules, listened to all the experts, and trusted that they would take care of me, that they were looking out for my best interest. I was wrong. Dead wrong. There is no telling where I would be now if I hadn't taken matters into my own hands, done my own research, and become my own advocate. It changed everything about the way I saw doctors and the medical system, and the way we have to operate within it to fight for our own rights, our own health, and for what we know needs to happen.

Looking back now, I can see how that experience changed me from a patient to an advocate, for myself and others. I realized that I had been passive and compliant in my health and healthcare. I had accepted the status quo of the medical system and allowed myself to be influenced by societal standards and beliefs without questioning the validity or viability of those beliefs. When those beliefs were put to the test, they failed miserably. It was not safe or smart to put myself completely into the hands of another fallible human, however well-meaning or well-trained. It was not advisable to trust 'research' and statistics that were given to me without questioning where the data came from and what special interests were involved in that information gathering.

Never again would I go into a doctor's appointment empty-handed. I went with purpose and intention. I knew what they could offer and provide within the western medical system... and what they could not. That shift in expectations altered my doctor-patient relationship. In truth, there were times when the doctors were not receptive to my information or questions. That was when I would look for another doctor who understood my goals of vital health and wellness. Not only was it important that I knew and applied this revelation, but I felt compelled to share it. I began interviewing patients and professionals in traditional and alternative healthcare, recording stories of courage, perseverance, hope, and resilience. Those interviews became the framework for an eye-opening, full-length film I directed and produced, called *Invisible Illness* featured on FMTV and Gaia, exposing the harsh reality of people doubting and even dismissing the pain of someone suffering from an invisible illness. Concurrently, I dove deep into the healing process and ancient traditions of Ayurveda, known as the art of living in harmony with self and nature, to become a certified Ayurvedic Health Advisor.

I would never have asked for this experience nor would I wish it on anyone else, but the value and impact of this understanding and being able to share it with you in hopes that it will change your experience makes it worth it. The value of shifting your perspective in a way that opens up new questions and concepts that you may not have previously contemplated could save your life or the life of a loved one. It certainly opened my heart to people that I would never have met if I had not endured these challenges. I would not trade those profound growth experiences and deep relationships for the world.

The most significant learning I gained from this encounter was never again would I allow myself to be silenced and submissive about my own body wisdom, and neither should you. Healing IS possible. Trust your intuition and let it guide you.

IGNITE ACTION STEPS

- **Listen** to your inner wisdom. Do not abandon yourself. You are the expert on your body. Start by connecting with others who have similar symptoms or issues.

- **Research** what you are experiencing and go into your meetings prepared. Do not give away your power by expecting a medical professional to have all the answers to your complex medical history.

- **Question** anything you don't understand. Speak up and ask more questions. Don't blindly accept diagnoses or follow instructions that are unclear.

- **Ask** for your complete medical records; look at the data and numbers. You have a right to information that tells you what is going on with your body.

- **Find** medical practitioners that will give you the time and attention you need. Fire anyone who refuses to honor your voice and listen to your concerns. If your doctors aren't listening, find new doctors.

- **Respect** the professionals, but enter any meeting as two experts with different expertise that can collaborate to find the best solution. They may be trained in medical modalities, but you are the expert on you, your body, and the conditions you experience.

Mystère Poème - United States
Director, "Invisible Illness" Film,
Certified Ayurvedic Health Advisor
www.mystere.life
⊙ mystere.life
◼ mystere.life
◼ mysterelife

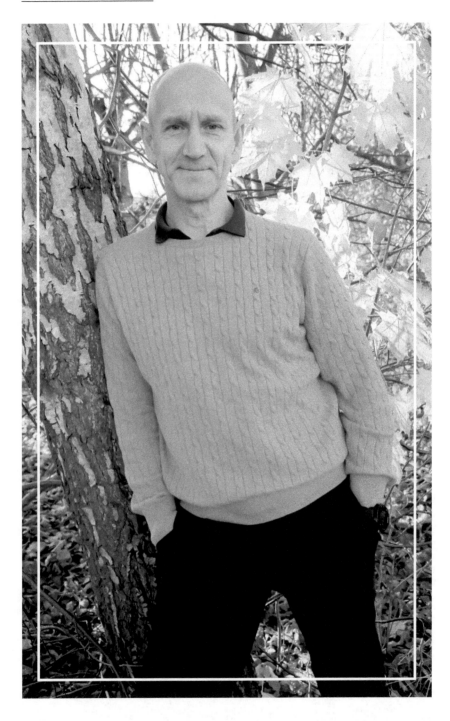

CLAES NERMARK

"Turn your challenge of health into an asset of wealth."

After reading my story, I hope you realize that a lot of your health and wellbeing is in your own hands. That you are inspired to take charge of your health and take it to a new amazing level.

MS (MULTIPLE SCLEROSIS) TO MS (MENTAL STRENGTH)

"Call an ambulance and get in straight away!" That's the reply I got from the operator when I called the hospital for emergency medical advice. I was shocked. Just minutes before, I was sitting in my chair at our dinner table, telling my wife and family how I could not see a doctor the next day, nor even early next week. I was too busy finishing off one job while simultaneously starting another. Taking time out because I was tired felt ridiculous. But, to calm my wife down, I agreed to make the call.

It was a Thursday night. I was transitioning from an administration job at a large Sports Club in the city of Malmö (the third largest in Sweden, and the capital of the south) to a start-up in holistic health education based in the beautiful summer holiday getaway of Halmstad. I was really excited by it. It was a real step up from what I had been doing before. I had two consecutive days carefully planned in order to finish off in style at the Sports Club as well as make the best possible preparations for my new job. The day before, I took the car for a 50-minute drive south from my home to Malmö and spent the morning in meetings, planning for my departure from the Sports Club. Afterwards, I was off to Halmstad. To save time, I bought lunch at the McDonalds drive through so I could eat in the car during the one-and-a-half hour drive from Malmo, past my home, and on to Halmstad. I spent the afternoon in creative meetings with the owners of the new start-up. Leaving those meetings, I felt energized. My brain was buzzing with lots of enthusiasm for my new challenge. I then drove the 40 minutes back home.

The following day was very similar to the day before. Car to Malmö in the morning for meetings, drive through lunch driving north, inspiring meetings all afternoon. But when I got on the freeway on my way back home, something was different. The two-lane freeway from yesterday suddenly had four lanes! Blinking and yawning didn't take the two extra lanes away. I knew I was tired after an intense week, but I did not have time for this. It was an annoyance. By turning my head 45 degrees to the right, I could *almost* focus and, as I only had a few turns off the freeway until I was home, I carefully threaded my way through traffic with my newly-acquired double vision. Yes, I now realize how crazy that sounds and that I wasn't a safe driver, but remember, I was sooooo busy.

When I sat down for our evening meal I told my wife about this 'weird' double vision that had appeared out of the blue. My wife was not as calm as I was, at least not on the inside. As my dear wife wasn't blinded by busyness, she very well remembered that I was diagnosed with a stroke eight years earlier, and she kindly asked me to see a doctor the next day. But as you remember I was too busy to do that. Luckily, she persisted. When I told her I was too busy, she cleverly asked me to call for some advice. As I figured it would just take a few minutes, I picked up the phone mainly to reassure her and told the nurse my current situation with double vision and my history of a stroke.

The nurse immediately told me, "Call an ambulance and get in!" In that moment, hearing the urgency in her voice, I saw my busyness in a new light. This was serious. I asked the nurse, "Is it ok if my wife drives me?" and she said an immediate, "Yes."

My wife was calm, yet efficient, and a few moments later, I found myself bundled into the car and on my way to the emergency room.

A few hours later, I met the emergency doctor who presented the results from blood work, X-rays and basic neurology tests, concluding they all were normal. I was given the option to go home and wait for a referral to an appointment for a Magnetic Resonance (MR) examination or stay the night at the hospital and wait to get in on a cancellation. By that time, I realized that I wouldn't be able to drive to work the next day or do any work on my computer, so I made the choice to stay the night in the hopes of being seen sooner. I wanted answers so I could get on with my life. After my stroke, it had taken weeks to start to figure things out, and I did not want a repeat of that waiting process.

Just before lunch the next day, there was a cancellation and I had my MR scan. Our youngest daughter and her boyfriend came to see me after school. While they were visiting, the doctor came back to give me my results. I probably should have been worried when he asked if we could talk in private, but instead, I sent the kids off with a hug as I was eager to know what had caused my problem.

"We found some active inflammations in your brain which is a clear indicator of a disease called Multiple Sclerosis or MS for short. With these biomarkers we need to do a lumbar puncture and some more bloodwork in order to exclude other diagnoses." As I had never met anyone with MS, it was just a name to me. I didn't feel scared. I was impatient as I waited to get the other tests done so they could decide how to treat me and get my vision back to normal. I didn't have time to be sick. I just wanted to get on with my busy schedule.

The blood work was done and the lumbar puncture went well, even if it was quite an unpleasant experience. The feeling of being scared hit me then as they had me hunch over to open up space between my vertebrae so they could push in the needle. I could not see what they were doing, but I could feel it. I kept as still as possible, hoping they would succeed on the first try. Hoping that all would be well. The preliminary diagnosis of MS was made the same evening.

My wife, Malin, had a very clear picture of MS as her grandmother had it. She had spent the last years of her life in a wheelchair before finally dying of it far too young. Having gone through that, my wife immediately scanned the market for books on the topic and ordered them all. As I could only read if I covered one of my eyes, it took both time and energy, so my wife read instead, telling me, "I'll read them all and if there's a good one I'll let you know and you can read it when you get better."

We have both worked a lot with mental training and visualization. There was no doubt for either of us that I would get better. This positivity spared me a lot of wasted energy. It also saved me from reading all the negative aspects of living with MS. Thanks to my wife, I had hope.

During my days at the hospital, with a patch over one eye, I googled MS and found an inspiring article about a Swedish singer-songwriter, Louise Hoffsten. She told her story of living with MS and keeping her career. This, too, gave me hope.

My wife kept reading voraciously, later telling me of faith-based healing stories or healing through cutting gluten out of your diet, but it wasn't until she found "Overcoming Multiple Sclerosis" by professor George Jelinek that she finally included me in her findings. This evidence-based guide to recovery with over 40 pages of research references, including a step-by-step guide, became my bible. I immediately implemented the program, adding flaxseed oil and a high dose of vitamin D3 to my days for starters. I wanted to take immediate action. I wanted to start *immediately*.

Three weeks into the program, I had my first appointment with an MS-nurse. She kindly and systematically described the two different disease-modifying drugs available to me back then. She said, "Both include self-injected shots daily or every third day and the vast majority of patients get flu-like symptoms three to five days per month. Most patients can live a normal life if they take painkillers in those few days." To make sure I understood her correctly, I asked, "Are you recommending me to take drugs daily that most likely will give me flu-like symptoms and lead to taking MORE drugs for a couple of days EVERY month, in order to feel as healthy as I do sitting in your office right now?"

She responded, "Yes, but the flu-like problems usually diminish after two to three years."

This was my Ignite moment. I sat there in that chair, staring at this well-intentioned woman who was trying to help. But, I knew deep down that drugs were not my answer. I knew what I wanted to do instead.

I kindly said, "No."

I wanted to first try to let my body heal with clean food and a balanced lifestyle. An all natural approach felt much more promising.

A month after my hospital stay, I had an appointment with the head neurologist at the hospital. Malin, having read all the science, came with me to the appointment to find out his view of these findings. The neurologist strongly recommended I start taking disease-modifying drugs. Malin politely asked him about the effect of saturated fats on MS and he said there wasn't any science behind it. When she tried to ask about high doses of vitamin D, he cut her short and exclaimed, "It's only drugs that have an effect on MS and the sooner you take them the better!"

I felt my first shadows of doubt. He was experienced in treating MS patients and as head of Neurology, he should know. But what about all those published studies in the book? What about all the other options? The all-natural ones?

Back home, my wife and I had a serious discussion about the choice I wanted to take. Since my vision was so much better, I decided to continue on my natural path with the lifestyle approach. I gradually added more parts of the lifestyle program, minimizing saturated fats and incorporating meditation into my daily routine. By August, my vision was back to normal and I was working full time at my new job and loving it. I felt fitter and stronger than ever.

Christmas Eve, my vision started to change once more. It started slowly, just a niggling thing, but the double vision was there and unmistakable. "No!" I felt scared that my lifestyle approach wasn't working after all. Was I back to square one? This truly dampened a lot of the holiday spirit as I worried about my future health.

The day after Boxing Day, I went back to the emergency ward. I managed to persuade the neurologist there to give me cortisone in tablets, as recommended in the *Overcoming MS* book. That way, we could stick to our plan of spending a few days in Stockholm over New Years with relatives instead of having to spend three days at the hospital getting it intravenously. Before we left, she asked me if I had seriously considered the disease-modifying drugs. Once again, I kindly declined.

Only three days into the cortisone treatment, my vision was getting better! At first it was hard to believe as it had taken many weeks to work before, but within a week, it was all back to normal. I was so excited! I took this shortened recovery time as proof that my lifestyle approach was effective.

Empowered from this experience, I stuck to my new lifestyle but, as I had some minor health challenges that might have been MS relapses, I was eager to learn more. Thanks to Google, I found out that they offered five day Overcoming MS retreats and I got us enrolled to the first one in Europe. The next summer we found ourselves with a group of amazing humans at a beautiful venue at an old abbey outside London together with George Jelinek and two other doctors. For five days and nights we immersed ourselves in the recovery program step by step.

As the motto of the organization is "Do whatever it takes!" it covered everything from disease-modifying drugs, diet and supplement, relaxation and meditation to physical exercise. All of it with reference to research findings and most of it as hands on experiences.

Equipped with even more tools and a loving network of support, I was convinced that I made the right decision taking the all-natural route to recovery. Back home, I tweaked a few more details from the program into my daily habits.

At the retreat we really bonded as a group and, before leaving the venue, an organizing committee was formed for a reunion. That group has had a reunion every spring since then in a wonderful manor house we found. Each event leaves me filled with gratitude for both being able to share my ideas, experience, and being able to connect with others. It's so encouraging to see the quality of life of all fellow MS'ers and follow their steps to recovery.

Modern medicine is wonderful and so much needed on so many occasions, but personally, I'm forever grateful that I found out that it's not the only way. It's only one alternative along with your own healing power when given a fair chance.

Just like chains I believe every body has its weakest link. When I put too much pressure on my body, as a result of poor lifestyle choices, it showed up as MS. I believe that by adopting a healthy and sustainable lifestyle, you can keep your chain strong and solid for a long, healthy and happy life.

Our bodies have tremendous power given the right circumstances. Without drugs, I've now been relapse free seven years and most of my bio-markers are well above average for my age. To me, nowadays, MS is short for Mental Strength, a gratitude and appreciation for all the learning I have gained since my diagnosis. As my grandmother Greta lived a long and happy life and, short of one week, got to celebrate her 104th birthday, I believe I have a fair share of great genes. Even though I gave my genes a rough ride for a number of years with a lousy lifestyle, I now visualize myself becoming "the crazy centenarian."

Your wellness journey begins with a single step. So, set your direction toward health and start taking those baby steps towards a healthier you. I wish you the best of luck and I hope you enjoy the ride as much as the final destination. You too can turn your challenge of health into an asset of wealth.

Ignite Action Steps

Crowd out. There's a fair chance that you, just like me and so many others, have set wonderful and life-changing New Year's resolutions and found them all crushed and broken within a few weeks into the new year. If you have to exclude something from your daily life e.g. "I can't eat x, y and z in order to…" is a common reason to fall off the wagon as you often end up with a feeling of lack or missing out. The antidote to this is crowding out. Try to add small positive and healthy changes one at a time until they become a habit. Instead of starting with cutting out chocolate, initially keep the chocolate but make sure you add a serving of leafy greens or an extra fruit every day. Next step could be adding a glass of fresh water to your meals. Next could be taking a daily 10 minute walk and slowly but surely your new habits will crowd out your old, less healthy habits one by one.

Start journaling. If you, like me, face a challenging diagnosis or situation, I recommend that you create a Health journal. Whenever you notice some change in your health, just write it in your journal as it is. Looking back in my Health journal, I could clearly see how my health improved from frequent doctor visits and relapses to my acquired high level of health and fitness. A Gratitude journal is an amazing tool to end those days of hardship when you feel stuck and just want to quit whatever track you're on. Take a blank journal and add the following heading on the first page. "Today I'm grateful for…" On the following lines, add shorts bullets with reasons for you to feel gratitude at that very moment. If you are unsure how to begin and live in a developed part of the world, you can start with these three sentences: 1) My heart has pumped blood through my body all day 2) I've had enough water and food to nourish my body. 3) I have shelter during the night. I prefer to write in my journal just before going to bed and that way I can end each day on a positive note.

This will will help you create an attitude of gratitude.

Claes Nermark - Sweden
Global Health Services Operations Lead Nordic
🔗 *claesnermark*

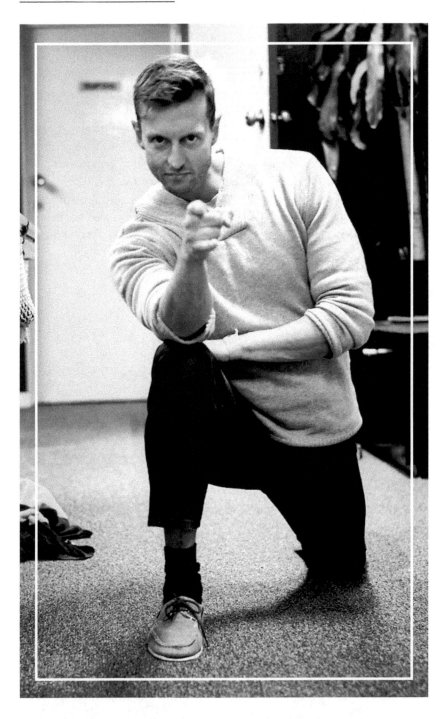

DR. BRYCE FLEMING

"If you think you can't, you won't... When you know you can, you already have."

It doesn't matter what qualifications you have, how many letters there are after your name or how many years you spend at university. What matters is that you can guide and support someone towards a genetically congruent lifestyle that supports mind and body. It's here that you find health, happiness and potential. Your ability to heal is far greater than you have been led to believe. Modern day science is supporting this. I share my story in the hope it will inspire you to overcome any obstacles that are holding you back, to have faith in your instincts and the understanding that you have the power to make changes that will lead to better health.

LIVING IN ALIGNMENT

When I was ten, I was the 'fat' kid. It wasn't due to neglect of any kind. My parents truly loved me. The problem was, they had a very limited understanding of nutrition, health and happiness. When they split up, Big Macs became an easy way for me to fill a void. I was one of only a handful of obese children in my area. I was the token fat kid, and I liked to do fat kid things. Video games were my specialty, indoors was my 'playground' and McDonalds™ was my Achilles' heel. Polishing off a Big Mac, large chips, large chicken nuggets and a Coke was a routine meal order. In fact, I distinctly remember crying and making a scene at the Mc-Counter when my mother refused to buy me a large Big Mac Meal… with an extra Big Mac!

Not only was my ten-year-old self too fat to feel like I belonged with the cool kids, school work didn't come easily enough for me to belong with the more academically-minded kids either. So I felt like I didn't belong anywhere.

Even doing regular kid stuff was difficult. I ran out of breath if I attempted to run anywhere. 'Cool kid' clothes never fit me and one of my biggest fears was swimming events and the thought of going shirtless. Completing homework felt as daunting as designing a NASA spaceship.

As my primary school years were coming to an end, I was excited about the new opportunities high school would present. I didn't want to be the guy who was picked on at school anymore. I didn't want to feel like the odd one out amongst my peers. High school was my ticket to looking and feeling different, my gateway to designing a new me and an opportunity to be like everyone else.

"Now is the time to reinvent yourself," my mother told me. It was a kind thought, but neither of us knew quite how to make that happen. The idea of inventing a whole new me was exciting and overwhelming at the same time. I wanted it so badly that it filled every waking moment of my mind, and I often found my breath catching painfully in my chest. I may have had no idea where to begin, but I was determined to try.

My best friend, the television, told me that 'to lose weight and be healthy,' you have to eat less fat and do long, boring workouts so that's what I did. I began conducting my own research (i.e., more television) and over the next few years I became quite savvy at low-fat conscious eating and jogging.

At the age of 14, I began applying my newfound health knowledge. I prepared and cooked my own meals and stopped eating McRubbish. I cut my caloric intake down to a small bowl of low-fat cereal for breakfast, a multigrain cheese and Vegemite sandwich for lunch, and plain low-fat pasta with boiled chicken breast for dinner. Within two months, I dropped an enormous amount of weight. So much weight, it sparked concern amongst my teachers, family members and almost everyone who knew me. The school even rang my parents, concerned that I was on drugs. But I didn't care; I was finally going to be a 'regular kid'... or so I thought.

By eating nutrient-poor food and exercising a lot, it was only a matter of time before illness struck. Colds and flus were frequent, as were doctor visits. My energy level crashed. I was angry, moody and irritable. I struggled to put on muscle. In addition to constipation and insomnia, my body ached with escalating pain. My dreams of being like everyone else were in jeopardy.

My doctor ordered a battery of diagnostic blood tests. I wondered how anything could be wrong. I was thin and doing all the 'right' things! The blood tests showed I had very low testosterone levels. An embarrassing examination of my testicles and an expensive brain scan ruled out a tumor but left the endocrinologist scratching his head. He couldn't explain why I was so low in testosterone so he wrote me a script for an anabolic steroid. He then looked directly into my eyes and with a calm yet authoritative voice politely suggested that I might not be able to have children when I was older.

I sat there in silence trying to process what I had just been told. As a teenage boy, not having children felt like a far-away possibility, but I was immediately taken aback by the suggestion that to regain my health, I needed to take a dangerous drug that bodybuilders use to bulk up. I felt so confused.

At no point during this diagnostic journey was I asked about my eating habits, exercise regimen or state of mind. However, these doctors were the 'experts' with years of medical training and obviously knew best — or so I thought.

I had a choice. Being a know-it-all teenager (and not being over excited with the thought of having to stick a large needle in my butt once a week), I decided to find another way and started doing my own research. By the end of high school (and after countless weight, health and self-esteem fluctuations), I'd amassed a small library of 'healthcare' knowledge and had decided that healthcare was the career for me.

There was a big problem with that career ambition. Entry into a health profession at most universities required 85 percent or more and after bumbling through high school, I limped in at 53. I called on my superpower — *determination* — and found a back door. I could gain entry to study for a Bachelor of Arts in Computer Science. At that point, my strategic objective became getting through the first year of my Computer Science course with a sufficiently high grade point average to qualify for a change to a health-science degree. And that's exactly what I did. However, I had no idea what kind of 'health expert' I wanted to be.

The strange thing was, as I recalled my health care experiences as a teenager, the idea of sitting behind a desk all day writing prescriptions for a waiting room full of snotty-nosed, miserable sick people reading out-of-date magazines and watching old soap opera reruns was far from appealing. I couldn't see myself sitting behind a desk all day writing prescriptions! I knew I needed to do something more hands-on and with higher energy! The Universe tends to provide when you are willing to listen.

I had my first chiropractic experience after sustaining a training injury. The chiropractor's office was modern and colorful; the chiropractor himself a tall, fit, cheerful man with a perpetually calming face. He took one look at my kinked neck, laid me on the table and repositioned the bones with a surprisingly comfortable 'adjustment.' Then with his calming and focused voice, he explained the importance of the nervous system and how it controls the body's capacity to heal.

This was a profound, life-altering event! Finally, I met someone who not only seemed happy with his work, but was also helping people to become healthy. The experience opened my eyes to my future and I decided to delve into the world of chiropractic.

It took me seven years to finish my five-year chiropractic degree. By the end of it, I was a confused pseudo-doctor who couldn't prescribe drugs; rather, I prescribed 'back cracks' to help with acute musculoskeletal aches and pains. Being pushed through the university system like sheep through a sheepgate, I was led to believe that my only role in healthcare was to numb lower back pain. It was made quite clear that I was not adequately equipped to help people with 'real' health issues.

As the years passed, I started to forget why I got into chiropractic in the first place. I was living and acting in a way that was incongruent with my core values and I'd lost track of my beliefs on supporting the body's natural self-healing properties. I became unhappy and began harboring feelings that I didn't belong... again.

No wonder my weight started to balloon and my health once again began to decline!

After graduating from university, I reached 108kgs (238lbs) — my heaviest point.

It wasn't until I moved away from the bustling city of Sydney, that I had my big 'aha' moment. A two-hour drive north led me straight into Newcastle with its many beaches and relaxed pace of life. There, I started working with a group of chiropractors who were absolutely inspirational. It was because of them that I realized the 'healthcare' industry I so desperately wanted to be a part of, was actually an industry of sickness.

The reality is, 'health experts' like me spend most of their time treating sickness because we know nothing about restoring health. Now I'm not saying medicine is bad. In fact, medicine has saved numerous lives when it comes to crisis care. If myself or someone in my family gets shot, contracts a serious infection or has a heart attack, I am eternally grateful that we have a system in place to save our lives. The issue is, we have adopted this crisis care model and applied it to ALL healthcare treatments. Got a symptom? Take a pill. Let's not address the primary cause!

Sarah Murdoch from the Murdoch Children's Research Institute in Melbourne stated, "This is the first generation of children where the parents will outlive their children… and all these diseases are preventable." This statement, although shocking, sparked a call to action in me. Under our current 'healthcare' system, we are getting sicker. It's costing us more and we are not really curing anything. We are always looking for something to 'cure cancer' or 'cure heart disease' or cure 'XYZ'. But are we really looking in the right places? Are the answers we seek really found in a pill?

I became fascinated with self-healing; it was almost an obsession. I started looking into the way people can have spontaneous remissions from life-threatening illnesses; why some people are vibrant and live up to 100 years while others don't; how culture and belief systems influence our physical being, and how that stacks up to our Westernized culture.

In my research, I came across the case of a 74-year-old woman who had initially been troubled by a rash that wouldn't go away. As time went on, things started to look bleak. Her lower right leg became covered in waxy lumps, eruptions of angry red and livid purple. Tests confirmed the diagnosis of carcinoma, a form of skin cancer.

The doctors assessed the situation and, given the spread of the tumors, determined that radiotherapy would not be effective, nor could they dig the tumors from the skin. "Amputation was perhaps the best option," said the patient's doctor at St James' Hospital, Dublin, "but at her age, she was unlikely to adapt well to a prosthetic limb." They decided to wait a little while as they weighed the options to determine the best case scenario for the patient.

Then, the "miracle" started. Despite receiving no treatment at all, the tumors were shrinking and shrivelling before everyone's eyes. "We watched for a period of a few months and the tumors just disappeared," reported her doctor. After 20 weeks, *the patient was cancer-free.* "There had been no doubt about her diagnosis," he said. "But now there was nothing in the biopsies or the scans." Somehow, she had healed herself of what is arguably our most feared disease.

"Everyone was thrilled, and a bit puzzled," her doctor stated. "It shows that it is possible for the body to clear cancer—even if it is incredibly rare."

Similarly, spectacular recoveries have now been recorded in many different kinds of cancer, including extremely aggressive forms. I find it most intriguing that many of these 'miracle' stories share a common thread—the patient's 'Belief.' When they had a clear conviction of the outcome they wanted, often their bodies responded favorably.

I started to do my own research and attended seminars by respected professors, scientists and thought leaders. I became a seminar junkie and loved it! It became clear to me that our mind-body connection is the key to being able to self heal. It may be our conscious mind that tells us what we should and shouldn't do, but it's our subconscious autonomic system (found in our brain and spinal cord) that coordinates the body's ability to heal. To be effective, both the body and the mind must be energetically 'aligned.'

Because our autonomic nervous system is so vital to human life and healing, our bodies have intelligently created a suit of armor which is designed to protect this system. It's our spine. What we are now finding is that restoring normal function to the spine actually influences the autonomic nervous system and the body's ability to handle stress so it can self-heal.

When you restore spinal function and support it with movement, nutrient-dense food and a belief in the body's ability to heal, it brings you closer to a genetically congruent lifestyle. That supports health, healing and improves your chances of overcoming anything that's out of balance in your life — especially your health. New science is backing up these concepts. Professor John Ratey, MD, in his book *Spark: The Revolutionary New Science of Exercise and the Brain,* outlines that proper movement patterns of the joints in our spine supercharge our brain, increase learning and development in children, and reduce stress hormones that are circulating in our body — improving our capacity for self-healing.

Over time I realized my time in Newcastle had run its course and I needed to take my new found knowledge back to Sydney. My wife and I started our company *Alignment Health.* We have a team of chiropractors, yoga teachers, nutritional coaches, personal trainers and meditation teachers all working in the same space with the same underlying philosophy: The body is designed to self-heal and self-regulate, and already contains all the ingredients required to be well. At *Alignment Health*, we supply the right physical, chemical and emotional ingredients; our clients' bodies do the healing.

I have been blessed to see people heal from some of the most devastating diagnoses. Myself, I'm now 78 kilograms (171 pounds). I am stronger than I have ever been, with a great physique, excess energy and plenty of testosterone. I have allowed my body to heal naturally without drugs, doctors or surgeries. I have never been happier or more self-confident. I also have two beautiful children and love my life. Career-wise, I have a very busy practice and enjoy speaking engagements that take me across the great continent of Australia. As a published author and TEDx presenter, I love sharing my knowledge and helping people to heal themselves.

The key message I'd like to share with you is this — when life throws you a curveball, have faith that you have an innate intelligence and a force inside you that is on your side. This intelligence is always trying to heal, repair and help you experience this amazing gift of life that we have been so blessed to be given. Nourish yourself with good nutrients and correct information and align your body and mind to experience life to the fullest.

IGNITE ACTION STEPS

Never give up. Above all else, persist. Visualize what you want and give thanks for already receiving it. The clearer the image, the more chance you will create it. Do this daily! Often, the best time to do this is in the shower. Combine visualizing what you want with powerful spinal movements: bending, twisting and moving your body side to side. Then, watch your thoughts become your reality. You can apply this to health, wealth, relationships, happiness — anything! You have the power. It's there waiting for you to call on it.

Dr Bryce Fleming - Australia
Chiropractor
www.alignmenthealth.com.au
⊙ drbrycefleming
⑅ drbrycefleming79

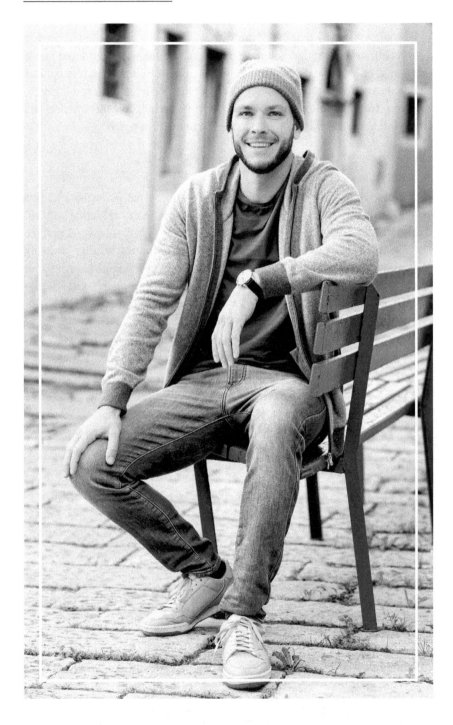

Maxime Šumberac

"Hard times are designed to make us grow."

I deeply wish that you will learn from my story and realize that health is a daily practice. That you will hopefully be inspired to pay the appropriate attention to keep the right balance to your body and mind, to see the experiences in your life as opportunities for learning and growth. Use my story as your inspiration; no need for heavy pain to make a conscious change.

Fighting with the Wrong Tools

I first saw the house on the internet. Something about the tumble-down pile of stone walls in the middle of the most beautiful landscape in Croatia caught my attention and I knew I had to go and see it in person. Once there, I saw that the stone walls stood naked and roofless in the middle of a field full of weeds and wildflowers, reminding me of a restaurant back in Montreal, Canada that had an open-air patio, bordered by the stone walls of an old building. Standing in the centre of the ancient pile of stones, I was determined to transform this ruin into something wonderful.

Nobody around me understood. Friends and family all told me that I was crazy, but I had a vision; I knew exactly what this place could become. A few close relatives tried to discourage me, telling me, "You'll NEVER do anything with it, that will take you over 10 years to restore, try to sell it, get rid of it..." But I had a plan.

Four years earlier at the age of 25, I was not nearly so hopeful. I was on my way back to France after a year spent in Canada. I had gone to the lovely old port city of Montreal to create a start-up that did not have the success I expected. There, I was surrounded by positive people, living in a penthouse with a huge sunbathing terrace where I would play tennis, far from any problems, and life was good. Later I would come to see it as an enjoyable life experience that I learned a lot from, as each failure is only a lesson that prepares you for the future; but at the time, I was not so positive.

Simultaneously, my clients and my former business partner in the real estate business were asking me to come back to Paris and it seemed logical to work again in this field, which I was familiar with. I returned to the Parisian dreariness and stress. I was financially in debt and now facing *multiple* pressures. The stress was extreme. The gloomy environment and negative people around me, as well as a huge mass of social charges and taxes to pay... I couldn't manage it all, and between working and long commutes, I neglected my well-being. I was like that old ruin of a house dealing with the impact of weather and seasons without anyone taking the time to care for it.

In other words, I was doing everything wrong. I had not thought about any outlets for the stress. It accumulated and bubbled up inside my enteric nervous system. With no way to express what I was experiencing, the pressure manifested quickly as an implosion. Yes... I mean a real implosion... real internal bleeding.

The stress had produced acidity and had ulcerated my digestive system, which was bleeding out. My body was so emotionally and energetically out of balance that I couldn't restore the order within myself. I tried really hard, I fought each day, but my general condition had deteriorated too much, the illness had spread, and there was no help on the horizon. At the time, I didn't know any 'real doctors,' acupuncturists, energy therapists, or other practitioners and my relatives were not educated on those topics either.

I was totally alone with this.

I went to the hospital repeatedly. Once, I almost fainted in the subway. My red blood cell level had drastically dropped and so had my weight. Whenever I was stressed, regardless of whether it was important or not, my intestines would instantly tighten and get more inflamed. That bad brain-gut connection pattern was well established. Every time I was thinking about not generating this bad process, my thoughts would connect to the organ instantly, and the inflammation would repeat itself, again and again... I was always on the verge of collapsing, but I forced myself to focus on the strength of my mind and my determination.

The psychological and visceral fear of inflammation grew day by day. Just getting out of bed in the morning had become a nightmare, with extreme stomach aches. Not to mention the mental trauma of feeling the inflammatory spiral that was spinning automatically in both my mind and organs. I was no longer the master of my own body.

Doctors in hospitals were still far from understanding the importance of my symptoms and far from having the knowledge to understand the underlying causes; they were administering vast quantities of strong drugs and antibiotics. It was not effective. I hardly had the strength to take a shower. It had become a challenge with the constant feeling of fainting, losing balance, and my physical weakness was affecting my state of mind.

Now, I know that it is vital to expel negative feelings and not remain under any kind of stress. Whether by shouting, crying, or using traditional Chinese medicine techniques, for example, you just need to get it out. Back then, without that knowledge and outside help, I kept fighting. I was struggling mentally against the symptoms, but the brain-gut connection had developed a deadly spiral created by a lousy mindset at a time of physical and mental weakness. I couldn't get back on track.

Unfortunately, I was not well cared for, nor well advised and eventually I had to go to the hospital for surgery. My face hollowed out, my tone was incredibly pale, I was exhausted... I prayed while waiting for that critical operation, that the doctors shared had quickly become life-threatening. I was hoping to emerge alive and in good condition.

Eight hours later I woke up on a hospital bed, immobilized, with no energy whatsoever, with multiple tubes coming out of my body linked to different medical equipment.

I have noticed that we are much more emotional when we are impaired. The people close to me who visited me, and more particularly my grandparents, were themselves in poor physical condition at the time, but they had made the trip from Croatia to see me. Feeling them shattered, affected, and crying... I burst into tears the moment they left the room. Being utterly helpless was a new experience, which left me no choice but to be in a state of deep humility that also pushed me to develop a strong sense of gratitude for the simplest things in life.

I realize that instead of worrying about avoiding stomach pain, not thinking about reversing this internal bleeding, I had to focus my energy on thinking about a state of total wellness in a healthy body. We attract what we think, and thinking about stopping a hemorrhage involves thinking about that hemorrhage, which means you are more likely to be drawn to it. You have to think about the result you are waiting for and not the actual process. Feel the state you want to be in. I had fought a lot using the wrong tools.

While lying in bed for a considerable period of time, I was reconnecting with some wonderful memories of my past that gave me beautiful and positive emotions, such as some baseball games and trips I had been able to share with my friends and teammates as a teenager. The fact that we exist for these life experiences, these beautiful shared moments, these strong emotions that remain, is what matters the most.

During my long recovery phase, I had to learn to stand up straight again, think about realigning my spine, and relearn how to walk. I had to strengthen all the muscles in my body and develop a warrior mentality.

Despite what the doctors said, I envisioned a full recovery! I was not going to let someone else's opinion of me become my reality. One step at a time, a visible improvement each day.

This condition had been a source of pain for me for almost two years of my life. I came out of it stronger and took a whole new life journey, learning a lot... a passion for traditional medicines, neuroscience, personal development, a connection to the Earth, and a broad curiosity with an open mind for learning, are now part of my daily life.

I have learned so much from this time of crisis, including the importance of getting the right information, accessing the right knowledge and the right people to help you overcome these kinds of circumstances, so that you can be prepared and know how to react and make the best choices at the right time. I deeply feel that I have today more tools to face and overcome these kinds of situations.

Thinking about it all takes my breath away and emphasizes the contemplation I had already made for myself, this gratitude for the "small things in life." This idea gets lost over time if you don't maintain it every day. When we become stronger or more successful, we tend to become prouder; our ego prevails in many situations and we forget gratitude. When I think back to this experience, I want to thank God for being today in good physical condition, in a positive environment, with a wonderful son, family and friends I can rely on.

All other aspects are secondary in the end and shouldn't influence my daily emotions.

My doctors had meant well with their recommendation of lifelong daily medications, an entire handful of pills each day, but I came to realize that they, too, have limiting beliefs that stem from their limited education. They do not have time to learn about life, the mind, how it works and the link between lifestyle, food, the environment, well-being, and new alternatives. After passing their medical exams, they move directly into the workforce, completely absorbed by the work they are required to do. Consequently, they do not have any time to question, to awaken.

When I first started working on restoring the old ruin of a house, everyone was quick to give me their 'prescription' for how to do it… or tell me it was hopeless and I should give up. I didn't listen. I knew in my heart that there was a better answer. It was the same with the treatment the doctors gave me: I knew the anti-inflammatory drugs that had been prescribed for the rest of my life would only have a disastrous effect on the rest of my organs, so I was brave enough to quit them in a progressive way, from eight to six, four then two then one per day, then not even one! It may seem like a trivial thing to stop taking a strong drug that doctors have said you should at all costs ingest at high doses for life in order to prevent the 'autoimmune disease' from reappearing. But, it is not. After all these trials and tribulations, I have overcome the fear they have tried to instill in me, followed my beliefs, and am very proud of it.

You should not allow others opinions to affect or destroy your goals, and this applies to all fields. The importance of words is also neglected continuously by the vast majority of doctors. They have no idea about the impact they will induce on their patients' mindset and their ability to recover. Every word remains anchored in your subconscious; every emotion it brings will remain associated with it. Each word can be salvific or destructive.

To protect yourself from absorbing negative ideas, you must stay strong in front of your environment. You must train your subconscious mind by filtering the positive information and rejecting the negative, wiping it completely from your mind so that its residues do not interfere with your thoughts, your patterns, and your general well-being. As a rule, you should at least say helpful and positive things about yourself, reassert who you are and what your strengths are, define yourself as the person you intend to become in the future. This process will help you to visualize that version of yourself and keep following this guideline until you get there.

Just as the doctors had instilled negatives in me, some of my friends and family did too when talking about my house project with me. All of those people are unable to make things happen because they live in fear and limited beliefs, and they would try to transfer those bad patterns to me. When I insisted on persisting, no one helped me. During this adventure, I had to face the many challenges on my own, but my mind was totally focused on following this plan. In the end, it only took me six months to rebuild my beautiful house! Then, those exact same people wanted to come and spend a vacation there and enjoy a nice barbecue by the pool. To me, those experiences are a perfect illustration that I have to trust my visions!

Ultimately this experience of rebuilding my house was unique. I learned so many valuable things, like setting my own objectives and doing what I have to do to get there. Every individual is unique; each person can redefine his or her own goals and accomplish them. There are no rules. The vision, persistence and determination I had were rewarded: the money came to me almost naturally at exactly the moment a new expense was incurred. It became clear to me that things flow to us when we have a strong defined plan and are committed to following it.

I have since adopted a healthy lifestyle with 'non-negotiable' and day-to-day practices.

Here are the elements to which I pay attention in order to be as healthy as possible: a deep night's sleep is crucial, sunbathing, following my circadian cycle, eating natural products, having a physical activity, and getting close to nature, letting the energy flow.

I also place a high priority on the way I start each day; my morning routine is rich and it evolves as I learn. It starts with dancing and shadow boxing in order to move the body's cells and create an optimal mood, meditation and visualization, a variety of breathing techniques, work out, Qigong practices that stimulate the immune system, making plans in alignment with my purpose in life. I have noticed it is important to set goals that are achievable. And above all, we must respect our own commitments. Adding a dose of satisfaction by going beyond our objectives is priceless, like setting a goal of 100 pushups in a row and then finishing with 102. Some call them 'small wins' and they foster your evolution. This method allows you to have a sense of pride in not only respecting your commitments but also going beyond them.

Renovating my house and turning it into a vacation-worthy destination was made possible by my unflagging belief that I could do whatever I set my mind to if I was clear in my intentions and my goals. Restoring my body to health was a similar journey of determination and vision. There are many things in your life that you can apply these same principles to. Ignore the naysayers. Keep your intention firmly in mind. Set your goals, respect them, and surpass them. Do this every day, day after day, and watch the magic unfold!

IGNITE ACTION STEPS

Be present, breathe.
Learn and experiment.
Get new knowledge, implement.
Set your goals and respect them.
Go beyond those goals and set new ones.

Follow up... I have noticed when I run outdoors during winter I found myself repeatedly feeling pleasure even when I saw that there was a storm outside. This could have been an excuse for most people, but not for me. I'm happy with these difficult circumstances because of the reward, and feeling of pride that becomes even greater. My run ends on purpose, with a steep and rocky hill for which I set myself objectives by pointing to a tree or a distant rock as the finish line, and I run beyond. I don't limit myself to running in the cold, wind and rain during the winter. Finishing that run, on the way down to the beach, I undress to gradually get into the cold sea water while breathing as slowly as possible and trying to keep control. I swim for two minutes while coming back with eight underwater fathoms, then I clean my breathing airways with salty water, I remain in the cold water and concentrate on my breathing while regulating my body temperature. When you force yourself to do things you don't like, you might end up surprising yourself starting to actually enjoy them. Your actions have a strong impact on your brain.

I used to hate the cold, so I decided to change that and took action. Now I love it.

Most people think I'm crazy to do this. I think they are crazy not to. You have to put your immune system under pressure; it's essential, with the heat, the cold, getting out of your comfort zone. Excessive modern comfort makes our bodies and minds weak. You must learn to challenge yourself, and you will experience the tremendous feeling of being more alive than ever as you emerge from that cold water with a new sense of exhilaration and charged energy.

Maxime Šumberac - France
Entrepreneur
◎ max_sumberac

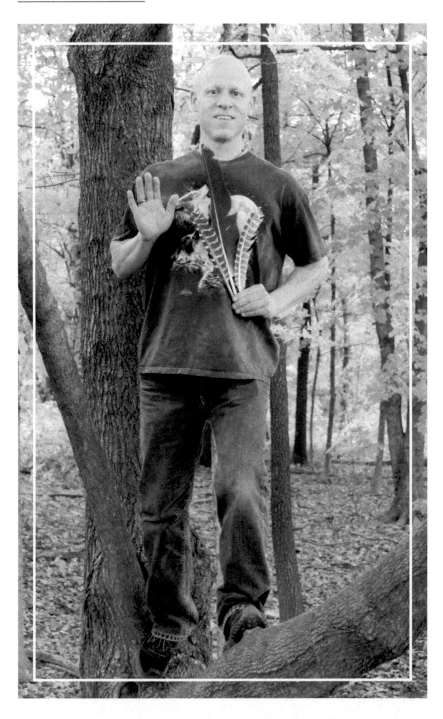

BEN IVANOWSKI

"The Most Potent Medicines: Love and Forgiveness."

May all who read this become aware that we are each creating our physical form from invisible intelligent 'stuff' which is constantly responding to our predominant thoughts and feelings. May you open yourself up to the possibility of self-healing by experimenting with doses of love and forgiveness.

RECLAIM YOUR HEALTH BY CHOOSING LOVE

I grew up in a nice little insulated part of South County, Saint Louis, Missouri in the Midwest of the USA in the 1970s. It was a typical suburban landscape with manicured parks and carefully planted trees and distantly friendly yet polite neighbors whose houses lined up row by row. In that artificially cultivated environment, I was taught, like everyone around me, to give my healing power over to the western medicine conglomerate. While surviving perpetual second-hand smoke from chimney smoking parents, I took aspirin and choked down cough syrup. When I suffered a skull fracture while hiking near Rockwoods Reservation at age seven, I was rushed to the emergency room. My skull was repaired and I survived an event so severe that it even required the ceremony of last rites. Not a bad system for addressing trauma.

Not long after that incident, my hair started falling out. I was exhibiting alopecia. Every time the wind played with my hair, I panicked, wondering if my bald spots were going to show. I was ashamed of my less than perfect appearance. Alopecia is one of those cases which falls into the catchall category of autoimmune diseases, a category that continues to expand because we don't know what else to do with mysterious cases. Well, it at least provides fertile soil for Pharma to create all manner of topicals and injections to temporarily mask the symptoms, but is it addressing the *cause*? Maybe there was something going on inside of me that was creating this mysterious pattern of expanding and contracting baldness patterns. There is always a cause and effect. The real challenge is identifying which is which.

In this universe of human life, we are constantly being presented with questions, almost like an alternating format exam. At the first glint of conscious awareness, I was posed with the same question all of us are posed with: "I am loved. True or False?" Since I was surrounded in the early days by the energy of fear rooted in a familial belief that a death prior to baptism would result in my eternal damnation, I answered, "False. How could I possibly be loved if I were going to go to hell before I was baptized?"

These formative years also involved a parallel path of Catholicism. Shortly after my birth, my parents stood up with the priest and my godparents to have me baptized. Over time, there was a progression of sacraments. I remember standing up as a young child in shiny polished shoes for my first communion and again for the rite of confirmation later as a young teen. I was forced to confess my sins to another human being, to believe that when I ate a piece of unleavened bread it was actually the body of Christ and then be confirmed into a higher level of indoctrination. I seriously doubted this system and I felt like I could not voice my feelings, but these beliefs were ritualized into my being by attending mass on school days and every Sunday with my family.

I learned from the modeling all around me how to monotonously drone prayers which seemed to have no real meaning, and how to stand, sit and kneel at the appropriate times. I didn't ever confess to the wine I snuck behind the scenes as a young altar boy; I mean it wasn't Jesus' blood yet. Most dominantly, I learned that I was separate from Divinity. That I needed a priest to be my intermediary within the church. That I needed Jesus to bridge the enormous gap between me and my Creator. Throughout this painful indoctrination, the prevailing and oppressive emotions were guilt and shame.

There have been many moments in my life that have 'shaken my snow globe.' Each of these moments could be an entire story unto themselves: being abused by the charismatic priest who led Catholic Campus Ministry, falling in love with a student-athlete and resigning my teaching and coaching positions from fear and shame, losing two close friends to astrocytoma and a young nephew to neuroblastoma, being open to healing work from my brother over the telephone at long distance to heal an injured knee, assigned a bullshit diagnosis of 'The Sweats' by a dermatologist, flung into fatherhood with the birth of an amazing boy, the decay of a marriage and a restlessness of spirit which is with me everyday.

Nothing rattled that snow globe more than when I picked up a book called *Natural Cures "They" Don't Want You to Know About* by Kevin Trudeau and became aware of my healing heart. My best friend was battling astrocytoma at the time — a long and ultimately futile journey through conventional medicine — and the book resonated with me deeply. In America, medicine is commensurate with pharmaceuticals. The book raised my awareness of how that plan plays out at multiple levels of control, and how much large organizations and the flow of money are involved. It showed me how there are so many more ways to achieve a better state of physical being than just popping a pill. Physical things introduced into the body have the potential to create wellness. Regrettably, when my dying friend called one day asking for McDonald's hamburger and fries, I delivered his desire rather than a lecture. I truly feel like I might have contributed to his early death.

Near the same time, I also read *Biology of Belief* by Bruce Lipton. This book is based on science that he conducted himself which renders currently accepted theories as incorrect. It also represents an upward path of expansion from just physical things creating physical changes. His fundamental ideas originate from his research of stem cells expressing themselves differently depending on the type of environment in which they were grown. He clearly established that there are powers more significant than simply genetic coding. For me, it provided a bridge into the study of quantum physics, how matter comes to be, the *observer effect* and so much of the wonder that occurs in the invisible world and how we can intervene at multiple levels to create a new physical reality for ourselves. This book expanded my awareness and my consciousness. Things that I *felt* like I knew now had a scientific explanation. It was a beautifully empowering and supportive awareness of how we are not predestined to any illness; we can intervene at any time. The loving nature of the Universe was becoming clear.

It was hard to reconcile love from Source with having lost a friend to cancer, but even more so with the life-shattering loss of my nephew. There are no words to express the pain we felt at my nephew's death. My brother suffered a loss that simply cannot be quantified. I decided to honor them by doing an Ironman triathlon. My wife created banners with the names of each person for each mile of the marathon so that I could focus on each individual. It was quite a cathartic experience of meditating on each person for each mile. The energy these banners reciprocated back to me helped to keep me moving forward to the finish line. I can still vividly remember 'going fishing' with my nephew Dawson on the last mile of Ironman Louisville 2011. Together, we 'reeled in' a lot of competitors on that last mile. I was truly inspired in that moment by something beyond myself. It was only later that I realized what I had been mourning in that Ironman was not only my loved ones but the damage caused by their unyielding faith in Western medicine.

I have always had a calling to be a healer, but since I was raised in a culture of dogma, capitalism and consumption, I also always had a desire to be really rich. Interestingly enough, this desire for wealth morphed and strengthened my truest calling. One of the simplest, yet most profound questions Bob Proctor likes to ask is, "Who are you?" Although he uses this question to thrust you into a new mindset about creating riches, it had an almost opposite effect on me. As I contemplated my higher self, I began to realize that I was far more than I ever understood and that, because of this fact, being rich was no longer my end game.

Another teacher of becoming rich, Joe Vitale, introduced me to Ho'opono-pono. It is a most beautiful 4-step prayer of forgiveness. Through Ho'oponopono, I can clear the negative data which has invaded my consciousness and restore a level of ease, returning closer to my true and divine nature. Again, although this teacher uses this idea for becoming successful, I used it to more deeply understand who I am and the implication of this process for self-healing. It is instrumental in the alchemy I am able to perform monthly when I am feeling the frustration of writing my child support check. It helps to transmute that frustration into the joy of being able to support my beloved boy. That is a miracle.

Choosing this path of investigating who I really am revealed an amazing sequence of teachers. When the student is ready, the teacher will appear. The people who began appearing in my life slowly solidified for me what had been a wobbly foundation. Louise Hay came into my life and helped me understand truths like "No negative condition can remain in our lives when we truly love and accept ourselves. Love is the healing power. Love dissolves anger. Love fades away fear. Love for ourselves is the power that heals us." To this day, I continue to work on expanding and broadening my foundation of self love. I also have borrowed many of her other affirmations, which speak to my struggles, and use them with a certain amount of discipline.

One of the greatest influences in my life comes from Dr. Wayne Dyer. On a long trip north to Michigan's Upper Peninsula, one of his audiobooks helped me reframe so much of the pain and loss I was experiencing. I was heading up north to visit my two husky hounds who had shared their lives with me for several years. I had given them up for adoption after my boy Stan entered into my life and I missed them terribly. Seeing them up north in the snowy landscape where they belonged was a delight, but a tangible reminder of the painful losses I had not yet processed. It wasn't just the loss of the free-spirited huskies, but also my friends and nephew to cancer, my mother and father within a year of one another, my marriage, and getting used to not having my son with me every day. Dr. Dyer's belief in connection to Source was so warming and comforting to me. He became like the sun, moon and stars to the sky of my consciousness. His conviction was like a massive vitamin B12 shot that gave me the strength to completely reframe my entire belief system and build it upon new emotions rather than guilt and shame.

I shared my growth and expansion process on social media. Admittedly, I did not handle it with a ton of grace. Most of my friends on social media are Christians and many of the things I wrote did not have a loving tone toward them. I was struggling to reinvent myself and establish a new paradigm beyond Christianity. However, there was enough truth in what I was writing to attract a handful of people into a private group that we called The Wolfpack of Spiritual Expansion. Within this group, we welcomed all manner of connecting to the Great Creative Intelligence.

One of the folks who followed me into this space was an old childhood neighbor and friend. At that time, she reached out to me for help with dealing with a spot that had been found on her lung after a consultation for pneumonia. I worked with her using several healing techniques. Without judgment or sadness, working from a space of kindness, I developed a mantra for her to use and meditate upon. A healthy lung is pink and spongy, a hollow impression of a tree with all its leafless branches and twigs growing upside down. She diligently visualized her lungs as being completely healthy and this raised her belief level around her personal healing. Her follow-up MRI revealed absolutely nothing to indicate any illness or disease. The best part is that she *continues* to use these techniques for daily health with great results.

As a renegade, I continued to push. Based on my knowledge of the Maharishi Effect, I suggested that we focus our group meditation on healing the spine of the child of one of our members. That condition could be traced back to birth, but was being treated via surgery. Many of us united in the ethers with our love and intention for the highest and greatest good of the child's spine. Our group member shared before and after photos of her child's spine with a dramatic change for the better; her backbone had changed physical form when no physical forces were exerted on her vertebrae. This event had a profound effect on all of us who were a part of it. We had intended kindness and support, with perhaps a little healing, and we created so much more. For some of us, it was disconcerting and disturbing, but for me, my spiritual snow globe had been given a good hard shake and it was beyond beautiful. I was elated at the dramatic healing effect we produced from our collective intentional direction of loving energy.

As my evolution continued, I became aware of a great shamanic teacher named Don Oscar Miro Quesada. I took his online course titled *Magic, Medicine and Mysticism*. It grounded me into the great work which has been performed by all indigenous peoples on planet Earth for tens of thousands of years. It is not a religion, rather an applied spirituality. A truly heartfelt exposure to Peruvian shamanism helped me to a deeper understanding of the soul's journey through one's mind, spirit and emotions, coalescing into a physical body. I learned how to playfully develop relationships with things we wouldn't normally consider as having consciousness, like rocks, trees and animals. A truly foundational concept of shamanism is that consciousness begets matter. For me, an effect of this course was an opening to a special relationship which I now hold with the Spirit of Hawk.

The Spirit of Hawk has been a guiding power in my life. It is medicine for me. It is a different type of healing. It is the true medicine that shows up to confirm that I am on the right track. It took some time for this relationship to evolve. I had to spend many years studying Hawk and learning how to spot Hawk as I made my way through life. It shows up when I am teaching my son a tough lesson. It materializes when I spend time having vibrant conversations with beloved friends, like another Ignite author who turned me onto this endeavor. I feel so strongly that you too could develop your own type of medicine unique to you and your situation, given time.

You cannot escape the law of cause and effect which is always governing the Universe. When an illness or disease presents itself to you, it is a great invitation for self-reflection, except for those with a victim mentality. The victim believes that things just happen to him or her, not that things happen justly. I'm careful in laying blame here. I'm not saying illness is a punishment; what I am saying is you have likely participated in the manifestation of your illness to some degree, whether it be a thought process, a feeling or a trauma, and you can intervene and create anew. When you move beyond victimhood to self-reflection, asking "How have I contributed to the situation?" it is in that moment that you can now do some work to change the outcome. We must always consider how we have contributed to some aspect of our lives which is no longer in ease. Or, by surrendering your ego and opening yourself up fully to Divine Love, you could invite yourself to be made whole again instantaneously.

And so it was that the alternating format exam of life unfolded and became seemingly more difficult over time. The true/false questions graduated to multiple-choice questions sometime in grade school. The age old strategy of choosing "C" or the longest response seemed to always be prudent. Then, fill in the blank came along and I actually had to provide my own answers from beliefs which I had memorized as truth. Matching questions were always fun. Short answers allowed for a bit more creativity. Crafting a response to an essay question allowed for the ultimate self-expression.

Perhaps the crowning question was saved until just recently. It was simply asking "Why?" It was in this moment that I realized this exam of life was just reflecting back my own beliefs, and that any answer I provided to any question was true for me in the heart of the Universe. Although I realize there probably is no "Why," it felt better to ask my own question back to the Universe, "Why not?" I returned to the first question on the exam and changed my answer to "True." In that moment of belief swapping, I changed the way I looked at the world and the whole world changed divinely.

May you choose to do the same, if it will serve you well. May you allow the Love of the Universe that is always flowing to you and through you to work miracle after miracle in your life for the highest and greatest good for yourself, seven generations and everyone involved. So mote it be…

IGNITE ACTION STEPS

- Read *You Can Heal Your Life* by Louise Hay and start your journey.

- Practice gratitude daily, as soon as you awaken, until you feel connected to your idea of Divinity.

- Practice Ho'oponopono prayer on a daily basis whenever you become aware of destructive feelings.

Ben Ivanowski - United States
Heart and Hawk Medicine Healer, Registered Nurse
Benivanowski@att.net

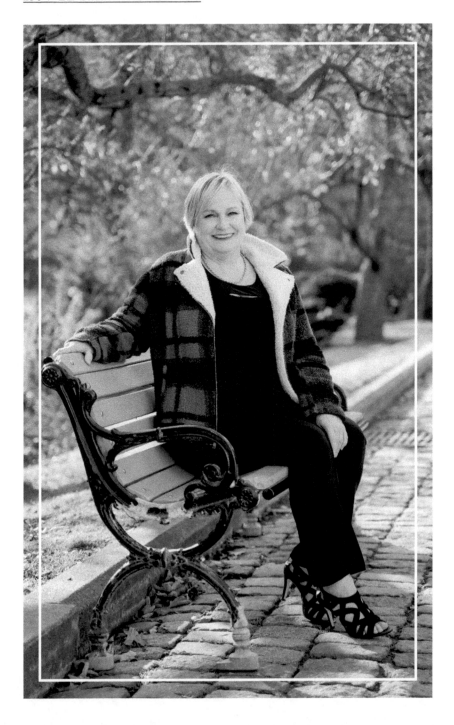

LL SAMANTHA LEGASSIE

"Never go over the hill; stay forever young in body and mind."

My intention is to dispel the 'Myth of Aging.' My story is of struggling to survive, persevering against life-altering pain, and refusing to accept that I was just getting old. This enabled me to discover the solution, a little known movement technique developed by Dr. Thomas Hanna in the 1980s called Somatics — and it changed my life. I want to share my knowledge so that it can change what you may have accepted for the future, no matter what your age. This simple relearning of a skill we were born with, and have forgotten, can end your pain. I wish to enable you to take back your life and health.

CHANGE WHAT IT MEANS TO AGE

I am only 56 and my life is over! I am unable to roll over in bed without excruciating pain; my right knee is swollen to twice its normal size, making walking unbearable. Stairs are out of the question. I feel like I am 100 years old and I am afraid to go outside in case I fall. If I do, I know I will never be able to get up and I will be a prisoner in my own home. Doctors are talking about disability and a wheelchair.

I am a single parent of a hardworking daughter who has just been accepted into the Masters program at university. She is only 22 and will have to quit school and take care of me. I will lose my home, car, everything if I give in and accept this. I must work!! I kept asking myself, "How did it come to this?"

In my twenties, I would get up in the morning and wonder why my lower back was sore. I was sleeping and relaxed all night, but my back felt tight and achy. Most of my friends were experiencing the same thing so I just thought it was normal. Sometimes I would feel burning in my muscles and I noticed changes in the way my feet looked.

I accepted the idea that my feet hurt at the end of the day, that my back would 'go out' and that minor aches and fleeting pains were to be expected. I believed this to be normal and, like everyone I knew, I just 'sucked it up' and carried on suffering in silence.

As we get older, we all suffer painful muscles somewhere in our bodies, but we ignore them. 'Never show pain' is what we are taught. I considered myself strong and capable and I would tell anyone who asked just that. I refused to accept the possibility that I was 'getting old.' Not me! Never! I refused to accept that I could be breaking down at age 30!

Three years later, I had a skiing accident. It was nothing spectacular... I simply slumped to the ground. I was embarrassed to be taken off the hill by the ski patrol, but my right knee was not in good shape. I sat in the lodge for the rest of the day waiting for my friends and suffering in silence!

The next day the doctor told me I would need to be on crutches for six weeks and if I was not careful, I may need surgery. I did not want surgery!

After about eight weeks, things seemed to be getting back to normal. Well, almost. I was not able to wear my beloved high heels for very long before my knee felt uncomfortable. As a ballroom dance instructor, I was not happy about having to wear flats.

Five years later and newly divorced, I decided to change careers and I became a Yoga Teacher. My years of dance had given me an increased knowledge of movement, but yoga was teaching me the importance of being aware of my body and its many sensations. This increased awareness opened my eyes to the subtle differences in my body. I noticed that the arch on my right foot was starting to fall and the muscles on my right calf appeared to be smaller than on the other leg. I wondered if this could be the dreaded 'loss of muscle mass' I had heard about, that happens to one's body over the age of forty. I had become aware of my body and its changes, but I had no idea what to do about it.

At the age of 42, I decided to take a job that would offer more financial stability for me and my eight-year-old daughter. It was very physical, long hours, heavy lifting, and a lot of walking, but I felt I was up to the task. For the first year on the job, every inch of my body hurt every day. But, I needed that job and I refused to give up. I did yoga and I got orthotics, which helped some, but I have to tell you that it was the sheer determination that got me through.

As the years went by, I was constantly aware of micro changes in my body's shape, numerous temporary pains all over, and tight and burning muscles that just would not relax. After ten years on the job, it finally happened... I fell! My toe caught on the edge of the platform and before I could catch myself, I slammed into the ground.

It was a bad fall onto both hands and knees. In that moment, a very powerful shock went up my spine, freezing me in position. I was unable to move. I was terrified! I stayed very still for a long time. No one could see me where I had fallen and I knew I was on my own. I couldn't even call out for help. Eventually, I managed to move enough so that I could roll over and very carefully lay on my back. I lay there for a long time, unable to move. I used my cell phone to call my supervisor and report that I had fallen, but I was in shock and still not aware of how serious it was. I decided to 'suck it up' and I slowly got up and very carefully made my way home.

The next morning was a rude awakening. My previously injured right knee was seriously damaged. For the next week, I experienced numerous recurring electric shocks up and down my spine, like the aftershocks of an earthquake. The paralyzing pain made me cry out in agony and my daughter feared I was suffering a heart attack. We were both terrified.

As a single parent, everything depended on me, so for the next four years, I fought tooth and nail to keep working. I did not want medication or surgery so I attended a Sports Medicine Clinic. I did EVERYTHING the doctors recommended. I did physio, chiropractic, yoga, massage, Pilates, orthotics, osteopathy, and even shock wave therapy. I spared no expense as I was desperate to recover and feel normal again.

All of my efforts were met with some measure of success, but nothing seemed to last for long and I continued to observe changes in my body. My neck and shoulders hurt now and I noticed that I looked hunched over. I just felt that I was getting worse every day.

It was now January of my fifty-sixth year. I had to accept that I was finished. I had done everything the doctors had asked of me, but surgery was not an acceptable option for me.

No longer able to work, I had hit a brick wall, and nothing would be the same. In that moment, I decided to stop struggling. That is when a strange calm came over me. I realized that I had to take matters into my own hands.

THIS IGNITED A FIRE IN ME. There had to be an answer to my problem! I decided to do my own research. Within hours, I discovered a book called *Somatics: Reawakening the Mind's Control of Movement, Flexibility, and Health* written by Dr. Thomas Hanna.

The ideas presented were medically sound and, most importantly, *logical*. I decided to order the book on Amazon. A few days after getting the book and applying the principles within, I was feeling changes in my pain and movement that had me thinking, "This stuff really works!" I felt hopeful — something I had not felt in a long time. I immediately decided that I needed to work with a certified Hanna Somatic Educator to heal myself and get back to work as soon as possible.

Returning to my computer, I discovered to my amazement that — at that time — there were no Hanna Somatic Educators where I lived in the city of Toronto or anywhere else in Canada. I quickly realized that in order to get the help I needed I was going to have to go to the Somatic Institute in Novato, California. That very day, I decided to become a Certified Hanna Somatic Educator and bring this learning to Canada not only to help myself but also to help others. It was a pivotal decision that changed the trajectory of my life in a million different ways.

I applied to be accepted to study at the Somatic Institute. Fortunately, my skills in ballroom dance and yoga got me in. It would require a time commitment of three years of study and a significant financial investment, but something deep inside me was shouting at me that this was the answer.

I arrived in Novato in the humid heat of August barely able to walk. On that first morning, as I hobbled to class, I did have a moment of panic. I had blindly pushed forward and risked everything to be here. What if this did not work?

By the end of the day, I KNEW that this was the answer I was searching for. What I learned that day changed my life... and I know it will change your life, too.

That day, I learned that Aging is a Myth.

We are born with a skill for survival called Sensory Motor Awareness that enables our brain to adapt and learn the necessary skills to survive — starting with how to roll over, sit, crawl, and eventually walk. Our Sensory Motor Awareness facilitates the brain's ability to learn how to control and coordinate the function of our muscles. The fresh new neural pathways that develop at this time allow us to enjoy pain-free, flexible, joyful movement and discovery.

Once we have achieved the ability to walk and run, our attention shifts to the world outside of ourselves, and we are encouraged to pay little attention to the sensations in our body. In fact, we are so distracted by the outside world that this awareness we were born with slowly starts to fade. We are told to "Be tough," "Don't be a baby," "Be brave," and we just suck up the discomfort and move on.

This is when our Sensory Motor Awareness starts to become Sensory Motor Amnesia.

With the passing of time, many factors start to affect the original learning and pathways we developed. One really important factor is how we use our body. Consider if you are right-handed or left. Think about what kind of sports you play. Consider how you sleep. When you are at work, do you spend a lot of time sitting or on your computer? Think about the ways you handle a lot of stress or how injuries may have affected your body. These are just a few of the factors that have a profound effect on our brain's need to adapt and rewire new pathways to facilitate the speed of action.

It is this rewiring and reorganization of muscle function and coordination that is the source of our muscle pain. Muscles that can't relax are no longer getting the proper signals from the brain. They stay tight, burning and eventually atrophying, which explains why we suffer the loss of muscle mass after age 40.

I am excited to tell you that the solution to our pain and suffering is a simple re-education.

That's right. It's brain work! It is a renewing of a forgotten sixth sense called *proprioception* that will enable you to regain those fresh neural pathways and erase the compensatory pathways that have taken over. It is a simple move-ment technique done with focus and attention to inner muscular sensations. Comprised of small physical micro-movements, it is relaxing and enjoyable and takes only twenty minutes a day. The results are astounding.

At the end of my first seminar, I arrived home able to go back to work full time. This definitely motivated me to do my practice! I continued to get better every day just by doing Somatics. What a feeling!

After three years of study my whole world had changed. I was completely pain free — something I had not experienced since my teens. I was not only a Certified Hanna Somatic Educator, but I was also an amazing example of the effects of this work.

Today at 62, the world is my oyster! Physically, I can do anything I want. I have even gone back to wearing high heels and ballroom dancing with an eye for competing again. I have no pain and no limitations! I have no physical restrictions of what I can do — be it jumping on a plane and hauling a suitcase or hanging from the CN Tower doing the Edge Walk.

My beautiful daughter has achieved her Ph.D and is a University Professor at the age of 28. I retired on my own terms from my old job and I now travel all over Canada teaching somatics and working to improve the lives of fellow Canadians and give hope to many people who are suffering with muscle pain and limited mobility.

Thinking outside of the box and finding a solution on my own was one of the most empowering events of my life. I discovered what I consider to be a miracle hidden in our own brain's abilities. I took action, did what I had to do to succeed, and now my life and future look awesome. At the beginning of my third act, I have limitless possibilities... and so will you.

Many of us are drinking the 'Koolaid' about aging with certain expectations and no idea of what to do. We accept that our body is getting 'old' versus knowing that age doesn't mean limitations. The body is designed to heal itself. Sensory-motor awareness is the one survival skill that humans are born with. Instead of dealing with the minor aches and pains when they are a whisper, we continue to ignore them until they become a scream. This is not a model that benefits our future.

You can improve and control your own future by redeveloping the skills you were born with through the Somatics philosophy, that aging is a myth. Our world would be a better place if we all refused to believe that aging is mandatory.

IGNITE ACTION STEPS

Here are a few simple methods to start to regain your Sensory Motor Awareness. The results of these actions will astonish and surprise you and help improve your sixth sense.

1. Close your eyes and sense that you are standing the way you naturally stand. Ask a friend to use your cell phone camera to take four pictures of you: front, back and both sides, left and right. Closely inspect the pictures for body symmetry. Notice what is your normal posture and what is off balance. Seeing yourself from all four angles will show you different body misalignments clearly. Use this information to help you see where you have compensations.

2. Ask a friend to do a short video of you walking away for about 20 feet, turning and walking back to the camera. When you watch the video, what do you see? Most people are very surprised at how they look when

walking. This recognition will help you make corrections for improved alignment.

3. Lie down on the floor and, with your eyes closed, think about how your body feels. Pay attention to the places that do not relax down to the floor immediately. They may relax after a few minutes on the floor, but 20 minutes after you stand back up, they tighten again. These are areas of compensation — muscles that your brain is not in control of. Doing this experiment will improve your awareness of where you need to relax and listen to the whispers.

4. Find a Certified Hanna Somatic Educator in your area and take back control of your pain, your body and your life!

LL Samantha Legassie - Canada
Certified Hanna Somatic Educator-(C.H.S.E.)
www.rejuvinagesomatics.ca
▶ *Somatic U*

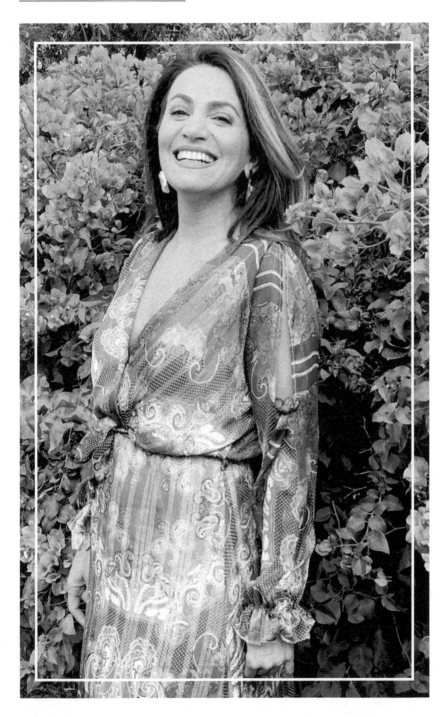

MARJAN TAVAKKOLIAN

"The bad is good. The good is good, so life is always good."

I hope my message can bring peace and contentment to your life. Happiness is truly cultivated from within. I choose to empower you with a positive and healthy attitude so you can live a peaceful and happy life. We are all responsible to make our world a better place.

HAPPY FROM WITHIN

Being from a Persian family and culture, it seemed like what mattered was to be rich and successful. The labels, the brand names, glamorous parties, high achieving children and of course, looking perfect all the time... was our way of life. You could be starving but you still had to drive a Mercedes Benz or BMW and wear (fake or real) Gucci or Chanel.

I lived in a 18,000 square foot mansion with an indoor pool and elevator. My life looked like a dream from the outside. I had what everyone works so hard to achieve. What every woman desperately wants to have in her marriage and lifestyle.

I did achieve all of those status markers and still felt miserable and unhealthy. My solar plexus was always in pain and I had horrible acid reflux. This affected my vocal cords and caused huge nodules on my laryngopharynx and made it very difficult to talk. My chest and throat were in constant pain. I didn't feel healthy or wholesome.

My life was surrounded by stressors, much of which originated from my relationship with my husband. I felt powerless and without a voice. Those stressors were so overwhelming that it got to a point where I literally did lose my voice. I could not speak both physically or emotionally and had to go to a speech therapist in order to learn how to use my vocal cords again. The amount of hopelessness that I was experiencing at that time in my life... there are no words to describe it.

There I was, surrounded by everything I was 'supposed' to want, interacting with people who had sizable status and wealth. Yet, the very core of me was lost and damaged. What's more, I felt the people around me were unable to express the least bit of empathy. To them, I had it all. No one understood the loneliness I was feeling. It was as if the world judged me by money and success. The exception to all of this was one remarkable man: my father.

He said to me, "You will get sick and you will not be healthy if you continue living in fear. You can go through 50 divorces and I will still love you and take you back in my arms and protect you forever."

He touched the core of my bruised and wounded heart at that moment. He understood the essence of my truth and gave me the confidence to start looking inside of myself for answers. He told me, "Life is very simple; just love what you do and be content with what you have." I was so scared of failing and ruining my reputation in my culture as this was already my second marriage. He assured me that people will talk no matter how you live, so the important thing is to be at peace and feel happy inside. I had the support of my mother as well and they both just wanted to see me healthy and happy.

A big moment for me was when our family traveled to a luxurious beach resort in Puerto Vallarta, Mexico with our friends. We stayed at a high-end resort that had not much to offer except for the name, very expensive food and some cabanas by the pool. I felt it was both bland and boring; soulless. Guests were not friendly and the atmosphere was stuck-up. Everywhere I looked, I saw people with attitude. My children, being children, walked through the adults-only pool one day by accident and were immediately chastised.

One day, in an effort to remove my mask of superficiality, I decided to be adventurous and take a four-wheel ATV with my son and few of the husbands and go to the local town. The ride was a blast with the wind in my face and the sun on my back. But what was even more amazing was seeing the people all enjoying themselves outdoors. There were big colorful umbrellas, vibrant patterned clothing and glasses filled to the rim with margaritas and piña coladas. The atmosphere was full of loud music, intoxicating laughter and dancing as many local Mexcian festivals are. I stood there, dumbfounded, watching these people with the simplest pleasures, having so much real fun. It left me feeling like I had been missing out on real authentic joy.

Money had never brought me happiness. It had brought me comfort and peace of mind but also expectations, judgment, competition and a never-ending pursuit for the next best thing. I had begged my husband to spend more time with me and our two children, so we could enjoy life together, go on adventures and live simply. But it always fell on deaf ears. He was driven to work hard to provide us with many material things, but we were craving his presence and a peaceful life.

I stood there that day, watching as people laughed, danced, celebrated and had so few worries on their minds. The connection between everyone was vibrant and the atmosphere was electric. Life seemed so simple and easy there. I knew I wanted that life. I was sick of the life I was living. Sick of the show off, competitive, ego driven, 'feeling sick all the time and never enough' world. Instead, I wanted to explore and be free to have amazing cultural adventures. To use my gifts to discover the world and help bring healing, connection and love. Witnessing that moment Ignited in me the awareness that I was living an unhealthy and fake life and needed to change.

After this trip, our materialistic lives became more firmly entrenched. We bought more things we didn't need. Another Ferrari, more homes…. Then, to my surprise, after the kid's soccer practice, my husband suddenly announced that we were going to get a divorce. I was shocked and completely taken by surprise as so were the kids. At the same time, I felt dark energy being lifted off of me. I had been too scared to ask for one myself, yet had known for a while that I wanted to leave the marriage, but I did not think I had the courage to go through with it for a second time. Even though I was sick and unhealthy all the time, I thought having the status quo was better for everyone, especially coming from a Middle Eastern family. And yet, it was not better. He asked because he could feel my cold and distant energy. I had been trapped in cowardice. My kids were young and I was hoping to remain together until they were out to college. The fear of tarnishing my reputation and upsetting my family was also very strong even though I always had the support of my father and his unconditional love.

Up till then, I had been seeing doctors for my chronic throat condition. The moment he mentioned the divorce and my heart agreed, my condition changed. Suddenly the intense pain subsided and my throat literally opened up that very moment and I was able to talk. I felt a huge sense of relief and both my husband and I knew this decision was the right thing. We hugged one another kindly knowing we would be great parents for our kids, but better individuals living apart.

That evening I spoke to my parents for hours without losing my voice. Little by little, my true self was awakening and my authentic voice was being restored. I knew FEAR was gone while love, hope and health was being restored into my life.

Since that date, I have been on an incredible journey towards peace, health and wellness. I have let go of my mansion, marriage, culture, religion, material stuff, expectations, a need for a partnership and having all the labels and status. I have peeled back the layers of life one layer at a time and it's been the most magical period of my life for which I am extremely grateful and feel blessed. I stepped full-hearted into finding happiness from within.

The first step after my divorce was to sign up for a Masters Program in Spiritual Psychology in Los Angeles. That two-year intensive program changed my life from the inside out. It became a visceral experience to go through a powerful spiritual shift along with 250 other students for two years. We were all in it together and we wanted deeper meaning to our lives. We wanted to meet like-minded individuals and grow spiritually together. Through this program, I was able to forgive my past and realize that we are all souls having a human experience. There is an earth school and a spiritual school and we need to be aware of both sets of lessons in our lives. In this program, I met incredible people and formed lifetime friendships with many. I also learned that most students practiced a yoga modality called Kundalini. I had the most profound experience after my first class. I saw colors and visions and the music made me feel like I was floating in another dimension.

Unfortunately, Kundalini is not a mainstream yoga practice so it was very hard to find a center in Orange County but I persisted and found a beautiful location in Laguna Beach where I have been going religiously for 10 years. The practice was so powerful and life changing that I decided to become a teacher and share this healing gift with the world. I studied intensely for nine full months to become a Certified Kundalini teacher and it has allowed me to divinely find both my chanting and my singing voice.

Kundalini works on strengthening the nervous system, by increasing body strength, promoting overall health as it touches the glandular, metabolic and nervous system. It opens up the energy vortex in our chakras as each holds specific dis-eases. By doing this practice, one can heal many of their ailments. The Kundalini music is pure magic as it uplifts and energizes you. Above all, it's a community of loving, kind, like-minded people who come together for the purpose of healing themselves and healing the world.

Many people I meet don't know about Kundalini Yoga. Yoga means 'to connect.' To connect to God, Light, Love, Divine energy… whatever you want to call it. It was never about becoming lean and muscular. I do Pilates and tennis to stay lean and fit, but I go to Kundalini for my SOUL and for a deep healing which in my opinion is like no other practice in the world. The intense breathing, chanting and the powerful postures are incredibly life changing. They have transformed me.

Through Kundalini, I continued seeing visions of majestic colors and shapes and movement. Even though I had never even picked up a brush in my life, I suddenly had a huge urge to start painting. I found an amazing teacher, John Eagle, and we started to do oil painting at his gallery in Laguna Beach. I loved our classes as John became a spiritual mentor teaching me how to be present, truly connect to the magic of nature and always grateful for the simple pleasures of life. We ended up going to Giverny, France and painted in Monet's house every night for an entire week. Eventually, I started selling my art in Laguna Beach. Today, I dedicate my time to doing pottery but continue to paint with mixed media. ART has been a critical part of my healing. When you create, you are in the moment. The power of NOW comes from doing something that releases your past or future. The focus becomes this moment. Nothing else matters except connecting to your heart. That is why the word ART is in the word HEART.

Today, I live a very simple life and travel extensively but very differently than I did before. My trips are about adventure, connecting to cultures and doing volunteer work in order to make a difference. I created a foundation called International Mother Earth Foundation which helps the underprivileged around the world. I have given up first class, I stay with locals often and love eating street food. I have moved to my dream town, Laguna Beach, and adore my community, my work, my art and my home. Both my kids are doing great at college and have grown up to be happy, healthy and successful human beings. I hold retreats and I help both individuals and groups to detox and rejuvenate through the practice of Kundalini yoga and art. I inspire and teach them to connect with their bodies, especially their chakras as each chakra holds an internal message for them. I absolutely love to cook healthy and delicious food. I am surrounded by the love of my friends, family, neighbors and a beautiful conscious community of artists and healers. How can it get any better than this!

My father has been my rock through all of it and continues to shower me with love and acceptance. His way of living showed me that being healthy IS the most important thing. Today, I trust my own voice and feel powerful to have my life back in my hands as I co-create with Spirit. I get to live and speak my truth because I know how terrifying it was to live in fear and sickness. I write in my diary, meditate daily and I never fail to attend a Kundalini class. Being in nature alone is another way I have been able to connect to my heart. There is so much magic as you awaken to the beauty of the world. Flowers, trees, birds, clouds, water… the list goes on. When you truly focus on appreciating the beauty around you, channels of love and joy open up in your body. In nature you hear messages from the Divine and feel inspired to create.

To have HOPE, FREEDOM and HEALTH is everything to me. It has brought me joy. It has brought me peace. I don't measure my success based on my material possessions, my title or how many followers I have (I don't even have any social media). Instead, I base my success on loving what I do every day and feeling healthy. I am happy from within because it is based on my connection to my soul and the trust I have for this divine energy that surrounds me all the time.

In the past 12 years, I have not been sick even once. No flu, no cold, no sore throat, no stomach ache, no headache… nothing at all. My throat and voice have never been better and my acid reflux issues are completely gone. When I look back, I am truly amazed. Every year, I am exposed to people who are ill, especially while traveling, but somehow I never get the bug. I even drank the tap water in India and didn't get sick. My energy is truly boundless.

I learned that living true to who I am healed all my ailments. It wasn't doctors and pills that fixed me, it was my desire to heal from within. As soon as I changed my life and removed myself from a toxic relationship and TRUSTED my *Sat nam* (meaning truth is my identity), my deep healing began. It was a total commitment and a lot of work, but worth every second of it. I know now that nothing else matters in life without my health.

My mantra is "How can it get any better than this?" And I truly believe that my life can't get any better than it is right now. When I talk to my angels and guides, I thank them for giving me this powerful faith and courage to live alone, travel the world and do the work in order to make the planet a better place, one person and one day at a time. I am grateful for all the lessons I have learned despite the ups and downs and I trust completely in divine timing for everything. My intention is to never chase anything in life. It is to be in the flow and just love who you are, what you do with no judgment or regret. I believe there is no right or wrong. Just love, gratitude and acceptance for all the good things and the bad things as it's all a lesson in the art of life.

Find your truth and do not fear the consequence as Spirit will hold your hand throughout the journey. Discover your *Sat nam* by truly quieting the mind and eliminating all the distractions of unnecessary things that do not serve your highest well being. Speak your authentic voice and then act upon it. Do what you say you are going to do. Live it, and be proud of it. Life is truly good. The bad is good, so life is always good.

IGNITE ACTION STEPS

- Find a Kundalini class and go without judging it and questioning it. Stick with it to find the essence of the teaching. It is there when you persevere.

- Meditate for 20 minutes a day as if it were part of your hygiene routine such as brushing your teeth. It isn't an additional; it is a must-do part of the day.

- Always use the mantra "How could it get any better than this?" Say this and allow your guides and angels to surprise you with even more. Even in bad times when you say this, the learning behind the lessons appears and you can feel yourself growing from it.

- Reduce time on social media. Focus on yourself and loving your own company and solitude instead of searching for outside validation.

- If you want something, use "I Am" statements. I am fit, I am wealthy, I am in love, I am healthy, etc…

- Walk alone in nature. Do not walk with a friend or listen to anything. Just enjoy the five senses in nature. See, do, smell, hear and taste it all.

Marjan Tavakkolian - Iran
Owner for Maison 38, Health and Wellness Consultant
www.maison38.com

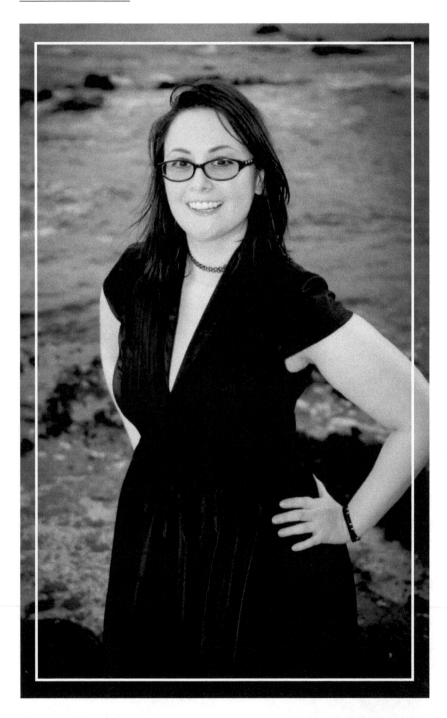

VERA MIRNA

"You will profit from this…"

My greatest wish in sharing this story is for you to know that you can bounce back from anything. Connect with my triumph and recognize that it is your absolute right to be the most powerful and abundant version of yourself. Your success is inevitable.

BOUNCING BACK: REALITY, RESET!

Physical abuse. Massive debt. Nervous breakdowns. These were the secret things that made up my life. But on the outside, I looked like a lucky princess who had just received my happy ending. I was finally able to get a job in my field. I was hired as a Marketing Director for an antiquities company that specialized in paranormal and occult curios. It allowed me to blend two of my biggest interests: business and the metaphysical.

My psychic gifts ignited being around clients and co-workers with such strong esoteric beliefs. The company's office was a playground full of mystical exploration, stockpiled with grimoires, spell books, ancient relics and haunted items. I used to walk through the office and feel goosebumps as I passed the eclectic objects.

My boss, Dee, trained me in the art of psychometry, the ability to receive intuitive information through physical touch. It was a very useful skill in the world of antiquities, as there were a lot of people trying to pass things off as an antique that were actually fake or very good replicas. My exceptional talent for psychometry helped us decide which items were worth researching and authenticating through traditional channels.

I remember one particular day when a customer dropped off what was believed to be a first-degree religious relic of a beloved saint for appraisal. Holding the object, my cheeks turned rosy and I became flushed with energy. I felt the deepest level of peace cradling this relic. I was so happy to be in a place where my psychic gifts were embraced.

As a teenager, it was quite the opposite. I grew up seeing things and hearing voices that other people didn't. My parents lacked the tools to help me. In their best attempts to understand me, they turned to modern medicine. I suffered through barrages of medical tests and weeks of being separated from my friends and family while under observation at a mental ward.

The doctors labeled me with a seizure disorder and put me on a heavy regimen of medication. They kept asking me if I was still seeing things and every time I answered truthfully, my dosage increased, along with side effects. I would daze out and drool on myself. The higher my dosage went, the less I was able to finish a complete sentence.

My brain stopped creating memories. There was no longer a sense of time. When people would ask me a question, I would respond instantly, but it would take minutes before the words would come out of my mouth. And even with all that medication, I was still hearing and seeing things. Part of me wanted to believe it was all real. There had to be some other answer, but everyone around me told me I was just seeking attention and trying to be special. I lost years of my life believing and thinking that I was crazy.

One day, I found myself compelled to research about seeing auras. I already had my neurologist's explanation of why I was seeing them, but there was always a part of me that was unsatisfied with that answer. Surely I could find someone on the internet who would have a better solution for me than taking pills and pretending nothing was wrong.

I found what I was looking for, people like me! Others who claimed to see auras and spirits as well. They embraced me through forums and chat rooms. I felt elated! One of my new acquaintances gave me an energy healing session and I felt like I had been born for the very first time. After building friendships with like-minded individuals who I was able to bare my heart and soul to, I eventually met one of them in person.

David was a charismatic flirt and everyone in our community loved him. He had been a professional energy worker for a long time, despite not being able to see or hear spirits. He attracted a lot of clients who claimed to be possessed and the transformations his clients experienced were astonishing. We started talking on the phone every day as he began asking for my opinion on difficult situations involving entities.

I soon became an integral part of his business, offering tarot card readings and other services to his clients. We had spent years being totally in sync. Unsurprisingly, a romantic relationship developed. At around the same time, I posted a video on YouTube™. This one video piqued the interest of Dee, the owner of the antiquities company, who offered me a job instantly. It seemed like overnight I had gained a career, a business full of clients, and a soulmate, while finally being celebrated and accepted for my unique skill set.

At work, my opinions and instincts were so valued that I was also asked to conduct paranormal investigations. David and I started getting paid to travel while exploring the unknown. We were approached by television producers who signed us and the rest of Dee's staff to create a reality TV show around our investigations and unique merchandise. Everyone felt on top of the world!

On the outside, everything seemed perfect. Yet, behind closed doors, it was the complete opposite. David was losing touch with reality and embracing his darker side. The longer I dated him, the more frequent and violent his outbursts grew. I was the only buffer between him and his eight-year-old daughter when she came to visit or while talking on the phone. When I reached out for help from my family, they didn't believe me. They found David so charming. Things deteriorated and I demanded David move out of my house. He refused. Without options, I started thinking about running away.

One night, without any provocation, David started to choke me. I didn't even try to fight back. My will to live had already been beaten out of me. Ironically, losing all hope in that moment is what kept me alive. He only stopped choking me because he was sure that my limp body was already dead.

He left the room and picked up a Bible. He came back in and inspected my body. I tried holding my breath, but could only play dead for so long. When he saw me breathe, he started to praise God. He adamantly believed that God had given him the power to raise the dead and that I was alive because of his faith. He refused to look at his behavior. Anyone who questioned him was evil in his eyes.

I didn't leave him, for fear of what would happen to his daughter if I did. I was constantly feeling overwhelmed because, as I discovered, I was an empath. It meant I couldn't discern if I was being attacked physically or psychically, as the energy was so thick and suffocating. Every time I was being yelled at, I would have a nosebleed. To help me work through this, I invested in healing sessions with a Reiki master. On one of the sessions, I couldn't hold back any longer. I told her everything, blurting out all the abuse I had been enduring.

"Please give me the strength to call the police," I begged her.

"Don't call the police!" she commanded. "His soul is in peril. He's been cursed by someone that was jealous of him. It's very dangerous, but I can break the curse for only $2,000." There were warning signs everywhere to not trust this Reiki healer. But I believed that a person who practiced Reiki and preached about karma wouldn't lie and create bad karma for themselves, so I paid her.

David did improve... for a few weeks, at least. His erratic behavior began again, so I questioned the Reiki healer about it. "One of his clients fell in love with him. When he told her he wasn't interested, she put a curse on him. This one is darker than the last one, so it will be $12,000 to break it," she demanded.

This pattern continued. Something bad would happen and the Reiki healer would adamantly swear on her soul that it required another large sum of money or else things would get worse and not even the police could save me. I prayed for a solution.

Things were getting worse at work as well. News came in from the reality television producers that there was no interest from the networks in airing our show. Dee fired me, as she no longer needed a large staff. David's past choices of not paying child support payments had made him a felon, so he decided to go on the run, taking our entire business with him. I was back to square one: single, career-less and client-less. The only difference was that this time I had depleted my savings and maxed out my credit cards. In addition to this, I had a bad case of post-traumatic stress disorder (PTSD) that made me afraid to leave the house.

Almost every night, I was having nightmares about the abuse, reminding me why I couldn't handle being touched by anyone anymore. The Reiki healer claimed to know the true source of my pain. "It seems that David was mad at you for giving up on him and not running away with him. He has cursed you. It's the most powerful curse I've ever seen. Getting rid of the curse will be $25,000 up front and $5,000 a month for as long as it takes. You will never be able to go to heaven if you have a curse like this tarnishing your soul. God will put you in hell. Because of the danger involved, you must not contact me while I am saving your soul. I will give you an update in six months."

I trusted her. After all, every time she had broken curses previously, I had felt the energy moving through her and I had seen the positive results in David, temporary as they were. "Spiritual people don't lie," I reminded myself. I borrowed everything I could from friends and family, took out loans and begged credit card companies for higher limits. Over two years, I put myself in over $250,000 worth of debt.

The time went by and I didn't feel any better. Obsession on how to bring in money took over my life and repelled any new potential clients. I needed to get more money in time for the next payment, but I was all out of ideas. I had already burned a lot of bridges with my loved ones. Then, an email popped into my inbox that I couldn't ignore. It was for a revolutionary abundance energy block clearing program from Christie Marie Sheldon. I was desperate to make this program work as my only other idea for how to get out of this mess was suicide.

As I worked through Christie's program, life started to make sense again. I had hope. My manifestations started to come online. A few people I had borrowed money from suddenly decided to forgive the loans. Others gifted me with furniture and necessities, helping me rebuild my life. For the first time, I knew I had finally found the real deal. Day by day, I was evolving. Christie did a clearing on emotional blackmail that felt like it lifted tons of garbage off of my soul.

"God is mad at you." The Reiki healer was back in contact with her usual pleasantries. "You didn't send last month's payment. Many people will get hurt because of you. That bad karma is all on you." I logged into Paypal and sent her the confirmation receipt of the payment she claimed to not have received. She tried to make up an excuse to keep her hooks in me. I was no longer interested in following a 'Guru' who required me to keep paying money in order to be repeatedly told what I bad person I was. I finally remembered that I was always worthy.

For the next few years, I devoted my time to learning how to deeply clear my own energetic blocks. I needed to understand how to do it for myself. I began successfully manifesting monetary windfalls, free luxury vacations, won a little money on a few lottery tickets and had a bunch of other financial wins. I had reversed most of my $250,000 debt, but there was still a little owing that I didn't know how to clear.

It was time to ask for a bit more help. I booked a session with Rann, a powerful healer, who was a frequent speaker on the energy healing telesummits that Christie had introduced me to. I shared with her the story of how I stupidly created over $250,000 in debt. I was expecting her to join me in a pity party, but her response shocked me. "Let's make it the best $250,000 you ever spent!"

"How?" I asked.

"Will that con-woman or anyone else ever be able to trick you again?" asked Rann.

"Hell no!" I shouted.

"That's right. Command the Universe that you will profit from this. You've received a valuable education on how not to be conned. You now know how to never be suckered or tricked again for the rest of your life," Rann explained. "What else needs to happen to make this the best investment in your education as possible?"

I sat with that question for years. The answer that finally popped into my head was my Ignite moment. My deepest desire was that I didn't want people to get taken advantage of in the way that I had. I saw that many of the legitimate healing tools had a high price tag attached to the classes and programs required to become a master. It was a big problem. The most desperate people weren't in a place where it was easy to invest the money required to do the inner work.

I continued to listen to the energy healing telesummits daily, waiting for someone to make things easier for all the people in dire straights asking for help who couldn't afford private sessions, but it didn't happen. That's when I realized: if nobody else was going to do it, then I guess I had to. I took every-thing I ever learned about energy healing, block clearing and manifestation, and made a list of the things necessary to create the world's fastest healing and manifestation tool. I took the items on the list and designed energy-encoded macros that automated the manifestation formula on activation and bypassed the steep learning curve of other modalities. I called it *Easy Button Healing.*

Easy Button Healing has only ten words to memorize in order for a person to master it. These ten special words make up three power phrases, where each phrase commands the Universe to do thousands of things on the speaker's behalf... automatically. Anyone can learn the *Easy Button Healing* method in under five minutes. So far, I've taught thousands of people how to use it for free, for everything from energetically purifying food to winning the lottery. Many love it so much that they are teaching others how to be the architects of their own reality and tap into their infinite inner power with this method.

My story empowered me to turn my situation into a blessing. Now it is your turn to claim your power and make every circumstance in your life a beneficial experience. Enjoy!

IGNITE ACTION STEPS

It is my honor to share with you *Easy Button Healing.* These three simple phrases are programmed with pure Source energy to clear out, bring in, and lock in place whatever you desire. You can say the phrases either out loud or in your head as you command the Universe to open doors for you to live your dream life.

- **The Clearing Tool: "Let's Clear That!"** When you say "Let's Clear That!" the programmed healing and clearing energy activates for the issue being addressed. For example, you could say "Everything in the way of me having _____, Let's Clear That!" or "What is at the root of my _____ issue?, Let's Clear That!"

- **The Creation Tool: "Let's Have That!"** When you say, "Let's Have That!" the programmed manifestation-pulling energy activates for the issue being addressed. For example, you could say "More abundance in the form of _____, Let's Have That!" or "My perfect _____ shows up for me now, Let's Have That!"

- **The Updating Tool: "Reality Reset! Thank You!"** When you say, "Reality Reset! Thank You!" all the previous energy work is sealed into your field. It resets your reality and gets everyone and everything connected to you updated to your new vibration.

I invite you to use these tools to instruct the Universe so that you can profit from anything. It's as easy as saying, with your strong intent, "I wonder how I will profit from this. Let's Have That! Anything that doesn't allow that, Let's Clear That! Reality Reset! Thank You!"

Vera Mirna - United States
Master Level Energy Healer and Founder of Easy Button Healing
www.veramirna.com
🅕 *veramirnahealing*

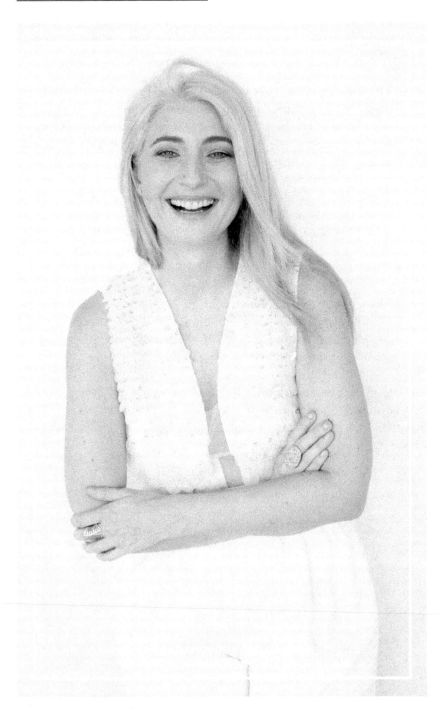

CASSANDRA FOX-PERCIVAL

"Go Find Your Happy and then follow it."

My intention is to show you "alternative medicines for the mind, body and soul." Something that opens your eyes, shows you the way, just enough that you can find it again later on your own. It's a combination of letting go of the old and bringing in the new. Find your freedom and you will discover your happiness.

PSYCHEDELIC HAPPY DANCE

Every experience, every step, every 'aha' moment is just part of life. There is no secret recipe, but there are Cliff Notes of other people's experiences and stories that can guide you in your journey. Here is a story of my life *outside the boxes...*

I had grown up the only child of a schizophrenic single mother. Our life was spent mostly running in fear of the demons that lived in my mother's head. We had a lovely home full of cats, but spent most of our nights sleeping in the car hiding from the 'bad' people. I had missed large amounts of school because it wasn't safe for me to go outside. Every day was an uphill battle. In order for me to survive inside the house, I needed to tiptoe like it was a war zone. And, to survive in the outside world, I needed to weave elaborate fake stories to make my mother look a little less crazy. The good news was I got very creative in my problem-solving capabilities and became a grandmaster at looking outside the box. The bad news was I had unconsciously been shown to never be happy, because it wasn't safe.

Well into my journey in life, the depression that I hadn't seen in a long time but knew like an old friend, came back hanging its heavy cloud over my head. A series of events one after another, over a few short months felt like an atomic bomb had happened. My father, my last living family member, had passed away, leaving me feeling utterly numb. My job, the center of my life for the last 10 years, had ended abruptly. And, my relationship of seven years had slowly crumbled to pieces. Life as I had known it had ended and I was left in an emotional haze with a broken heart.

For days, I really didn't feel the need to live anymore. My face hung in sadness, my eyes stung with tears, my heart was in constant pain. I couldn't move off the sofa. If I was lucky I could manage to go take a shower and lay on the floor in there, for a change of scenery. I closed myself off from the world and hid in my box of safety.

Finally, one of my friends called to check on me. I tried to be strong and stoic and I failed miserably, crumbling in tears over the phone. She said, "Cassie, you can do this." I said, "No, No, I can't." She was the first of many people who picked up my disheveled pieces, brushed me off and told me I would be okay. She believed in me when I didn't believe in myself. "Cassie, go to India," she said. "Write a book about it. You like to write. Share your stories so the next person doesn't have to suffer as much as you have." She gave hope when mine was all but depleted.

I thought, "Yeah… maybe I could do that." It was like she had given me a homework assignment and, in that *Ignite* moment, it became my reason to put one foot in front of the other. Searching for meaning, I decided I *would* go find myself in India. I gave myself three weeks because that was surely enough time to find oneself.

Eventually, this commitment to helping the next person became my permission to live vicariously for them. I travelled the world having the most amazing experiences because I was writing a book about it. I gave myself permission to do many things I never would have tried, because it would make a good chapter in my book. I rode elephants in India, meditated with Gurus in the Himalayas, salsa danced in Cuba, even attended a swingers party for fun in Rio de Janeiro, Brazil. How amazing would this world be if we all lived our lives so vibrantly we could write a book about it?

I still haven't found what I was looking for, but what an amazing adventure

I have had! Just like life, it's not where you're going, it's how much fun you have between now and then.

Here are my 'Out of the Box' stories to help open your eyes to new things. Life is a blank canvas, collect what you need and leave the rest behind. Sometimes the best decisions in my life had nothing to do with me. I blindly followed, most of the time with heavy, non-believing feet, but I am so thankful I did.

Freedom in dance

In India, I danced my way to freedom. I had never in my life danced, but three minutes of ecstatic dance in the middle of the India hilltops and I found joy. Dancing, jumping, singing... I tried to recollect the last time I felt that way; it must have been when I was still just a child.

We can all dance. It's a freedom that comes with releasing control and letting your body do what it wants. A freedom that, when I found it, I did not have but I so desperately needed. Dance is a time to let go, to not think, to let life's tensions fall away.

My hands slowly fly like birds through the sky. I move where it feels good. I am stretching, reminding, remembering. The hips go where they want. I inhale. Happiness flows in me. I smile. I remember. I breathe deeper letting the air fill me. The distance between my soul and the music is getting smaller. Waiting for the moment when we become one.

I danced my way around the world in sunset meditations as my back-drop in beautiful places like Greece and Spain. I took that freedom of dance with me wherever I went. People watched while I danced, but then I started noticing they danced too. The wake of my search for happiness was inspiring people I didn't even know.

Next came Havana, Cuba, and salsa. Previously what I would have called a deep intimate relationship, Latinos would call dancing. In America, we do things like shake hands, live in big houses, drive our own cars... anything that gives us space. On my first day of Reggaeton class, I was sure that I had never in my life stood so close to a man, especially one I didn't know. The top of his fluffy hair came just about to my chin. I could smell his shampoo, his skin, even get lost in his perfume. We stood so close I started to ponder about silly things, like what I ate for breakfast or did I brush my teeth this morning?

The first few weeks in Cuba, my eyes were in a constant state of surprise.

Everything I saw there I had never seen before. I would stop and watch a couple dancing in the street to live music. It was so sexy, romantic, perfect, and absolutely breathtaking. I would think to myself, wow what a beautiful couple. Then the music would stop and they would walk away from each other in opposite directions. Complete strangers. My mind was blown.

I stayed in Cuba for three months, learning how to salsa dance. I was like a kid in a candy store. Living in this colorful, vibrant city everyday. The best part, I was a beginner all over again. I learned about music, rhythm, listening, timing, leading, following, sensuality, grace and *Sabrosura*. All things I could learn and later put back into my own teaching. I discovered things about my body that I had never really bothered to look at so closely before. How to move this part or that part of the body was really so fascinating and surprisingly hard.

Dancing ignited in me freedom to let go and be me.

Meditation through movement

When my therapist found out I was going to be moving to Thailand, she told me, "Cassie, Thailand is the best place to learn how to meditate. Promise me you will try it." So I promised, and then I tried. I learned meditation from a monk at a temple near my home. Every morning, I sat at his feet and we meditated together: *Breathing In, Breathing Out*. Hours, days, and months passed with us like this. My weekends were spent listening to spiritual gurus give inspirational talks and I went on 10-day Silent Vipassana retreats. On the outside, it was a recipe for success as I had been taught by the best gurus in the most ideal place on earth. Yet, somehow, 10 years passed by and I never really understood what all the hype with meditation was about, until later in India, I accidentally found a new kind of dancing meditation by Osho. They were active meditations aimed at taming the fast paced foreigner's mind and worked much better for me. This was the first time I actually saw there was hope for meditation changing my life. I spent three months, eight hours a day hiding in the hilltops of Rishikesh, India learning to meditate. It was a simple switch in my head. Osho for me opened my eyes to possibilities in the meditation world that I would have never known were there, had I not gone out of the box and followed the Universe blindly.

Meditation ignited in me the willingness to surrender and be more of me.

The Psychedelic Happy Dance

I have been a late bloomer in just about everything I have done. I didn't have my first kiss until I was 21, or my first drink until 22 and lost my virginity at the ripe old age of 25. So, it is no wonder that when most people were experimenting with drugs in college I didn't even get to them until nearly a decade later. The good news is that as we get older, we develop a curiosity about why things are the way they are and how they can help us better ourselves. Until about three years ago, I had never in my life done a drug. Thanks to a boyfriend in India that all changed. I admit my reasons for trying was wanting to be a little misbehaved and break free from the life as I had known it, but what I got in return was the most beautiful gift I could have imagined.

What people don't realize is that Psychedelics have the ability to enhance the mind, free the soul, guide the spirit, make us dance and remind us how to love, when used wisely. They have the innate ability to break down walls that have been built up over the years due to self-consciousness, worry, fear, social anxiety and depression. In return, life becomes this beautiful place we suddenly feel deeply connected with. Healing through Psychedelics has been the most amazing experience of my life.

I have had my fair share of therapy... eight years to be exact. Although most of it was helpful at the time, I found many years later I had deeper, faster breakthroughs taking Psychedelics. Most prescription drugs given by therapists lessen symptoms for things like depression, social anxiety, and PTSD, but they often take a long time to get to the root of the problem.

Psychedelics, on the other hand, let a person's mind process what it needs, when it needs. Individuals can see and have the experiences They are supposed to have. Problems often don't even seem problems anymore. The Ego takes a backseat, allowing One to be completely free, happy, understanding, compassionate and love all in the blink of an eye.

In Portugal, my first time on 'Molls', the world curved around me like I was in my own little snow globe. I could reach out, touch the stars, lay my hat on the moon, and kiss my lover with my feet in the sand, while the music echoed through the air around us

In Mexico, on 'Zen', I sat with my friend on matching lounge chairs happily watching the world go by like it was a movie. I had never in my life laughed so hard. We lay literally glued to our chairs in fits of laughter. Hours later, we made it to the sand where I sat, reflective about life. Imagining with each breath I controlled the waves of the ocean. Breathing in, Breathing out. How could I have never noticed how beautiful sand was before? The jungle trees hung low over our heads, plump with furry green voluptuous leaves vibrating with energy.

In the Netherlands, on 'shrooms', I sat in my friend's yard, both of us giggling like children. Watching his tiny dead garden of weeds dance in the wind. The most beautiful thing I had ever seen. Every time I breathed, I was filled with this overwhelming sense of love from this plant. We exchanged feelings when there were not words. I wanted to cry. I felt how beautiful this world is we live in and how lucky was I to get to experience this.

My experience with 'Toad' flashed me to heaven for maybe a few seconds, but it was enough. The music played as I floated in the Technicolor universe, so breathtakingly beautiful. I giggled at the overwhelming feeling of love all around me. I was love. A feeling so amazing no words will ever do it justice.

Those moments ignited in me more joy and bliss.

I came to this realization that humans and the spiritual world are just separated by a little blanket in the sky. A blanket that you can reach up and peel away anytime you like. We begin to realize we can play between these worlds. I believe that this planet is our playground and we all have chosen to play the game of Life here. I started wanting to make this world a better place by spreading happiness and smiles everywhere I went.

We as a human race are all just trying to heal ourselves, as fast as possible so we can live our best lives. I want to live my life vibrantly and fully. And I want you to do the same. We are all people, on different journeys to the same place. I encourage you to try as many things *outside the box* as you can. Keep looking, searching and trying to find what serves your soul the best. Something that opens your eyes to new possibilities. Don't live a life of suffering because what worked for other people didn't work for you. If you never try you will never know. We, humans, are constantly in a state of building a better version of ourselves.

Don't live a blah uninteresting life because it's easy. Feel free to walk blindly into situations you don't understand because you are looking for something. Even if you're not quite sure what that is, sometimes showing up is enough. Some people call it hope, some people call it God, some people call it the Universe. But just know whatever you believe in, It has your back. You will always have the experiences you're supposed to have and meet the people you are supposed to meet. This is your life, there is only one of you and there are no rules. Don't lead your life by other people's expectations; just follow your heart one leap or one tip-toe at a time. Be kind, be free and Live in the moment. Spread joy, give love and remember you are a gift to every room you walk into.

Ignite Action Steps

- Find someone who makes you feel good to be around, lets you be you, and is intrigued by your wisdom. Surround yourself with people that serve you in your journey now. Let go of the friends that don't serve you anymore, and new ones will arrive.

- Go Find Your Happy and then follow it. Don't let yourself forget how to be happy. How to smile. Laugh genuinely. Belly laugh uncontrollably like a child as often as possible.

- Morning gratitude. Take three minutes before you get out of bed to go through your day yesterday and think of all the things that happened that you have gratitude for. Remember how it made you feel. It is a practice that will create more.

- DANCE meditation. Take five minutes to turn on the music and DANCE! Feel free, happy, alive, and sexy.

- Do as many things 'outside the box' as you can. Keep looking, searching and finding what serves your soul the best and opens your eyes to new possibilities.

You have gone, come back, conquered, bowed down, understood, asked, answered, loved, been compassionate, had freedom, followed, led, saved, surrendered, seen the world, flown in the universe, loved the plants, inhaled, exhaled, and then calmly been put back in your body. Welcome back to earth my friend. You are now ready to be human again, please proceed with kindness, compassion and understanding.

Cassandra Fox-Percival - Thailand
Classical Musician, Joy Giver, Happiness Finder
cassieaf@gmail.com

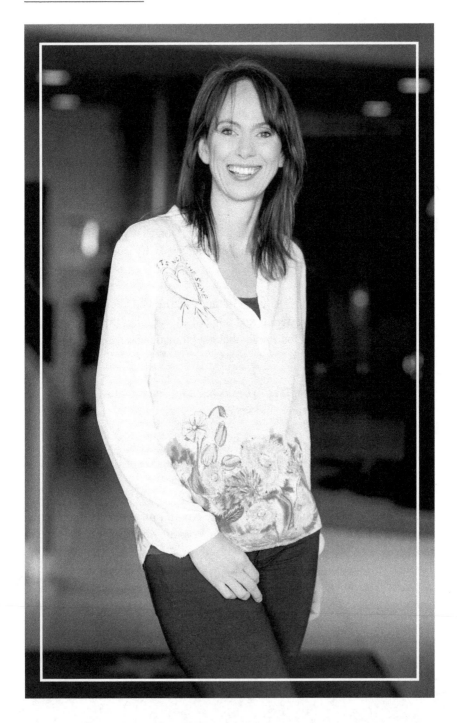

HILDE JAHREN

"Change can only happen when you do something different."

My intention is to help you realize that there is nothing wrong with you. I want you to disregard those who are saying otherwise, including your own voice! You are NOT broken, my dear. You are not a lost case. You are ENOUGH. When you decide you want a change and have found your WHY for doing it, anything is possible.

THEN WE BROKE UP – MY SUGAR AND I

"Mind your own business and stop questioning me… those are MINE!!! You have NO right to sneak up on me and then try to take them away!" I yelled at my son. "Just leave me alone; go do something else!"

At first, my son was standing peacefully in the kitchen having just observed me secretly reaching for my hidden sweets when I thought no one would catch me. Kindly, he had said to me, "I think it is smart if I take away your sweets for a little while Mum as I can clearly see that they are not good for you anymore." This beautiful soul… who loves me. I'm his mama and he had observed me over time, feeling my moods, my low energy, my grumpiness and my stress. Now, he was looking at me with wide open eyes, worried and scared, "What is going on Mum? Why are you acting this way? Calm down please…"

I had just snapped at him, my own son, because I felt threatened by his wanting to take away my rescue, my precious, my candy. My face heated with a rush of guilt and shame that came over me. How could I as a mother behave in this way? How did I end up in this situation? I was NOT handling this well, a caring act from my son, and the guilt of it lay heavily on my heart. I felt shame for using the candies as a rescue and showing my children how NOT to be. I stared at the floor, frustrated for suddenly discovering I was a little tantrum-girl and my son had taken on the parenting role. This was not how I wanted to lead my life!

I asked for forgiveness and we moved on to have dinner. As I ate my meal, my sadness was heavily lingering.

Earlier that day, I had been busy at work, as usual, having the all-too-well-known feeling of stress hovering over me, haunting me like the plague, constantly hanging around making me feel less worthy, not good enough and exhausted. I struggled to focus or to complete things on time and it was in one of these brain fog moments that I turned to my quick fix, "Sweets, please rescue me."

I hid my sweets away in my drawers, handbags, cupboards, pockets and in the car. No one could know about my treats. I was supposed to be the smart and healthy one. Having to hide this from my family and friends for fear of my unhealthy addiction being found out was just too embarrassing. My sweet things were my go-to, 'my precious.'

The sweets were like my perfect 'life partner;' they didn't ask anything of me, didn't demand my time or become a point on my to-do-list. In retrospect though, they *did* demand my energy, a lot of it, but I wasn't willing to look at that then.

We rushed through dinner that night and then I took my kids to their various activities. At their lessons, I could feel the muscles in my neck tensing up with the knowledge that I needed to go back to work as deadlines were approaching. Later, as I said good night to my boys, they asked why I was going back to work that night... *again*. They asked, "Did I not want to be with them?" Like so many evenings I worked late into the night after my mommy-duties. *They* wanted me home. Oh, man! That was like a punch in my stomach! It was so painful; the mama-guilt was bleeding wide open. It was the exact opposite of what I wanted to do, but I felt stuck in a rut. I was struggling to be focused and effective at work, and all the long nights took more out of me than I was willing to admit.

Back at my desk, I felt so sorry for myself. As I and many of us often do, I wanted to blame my misery on my tough circumstances, just pitying myself.

So what does a lady do? She comforts herself with some sweets! I believed that sugar was the only thing that could 'help' me and keep me awake so that I was able to stay working. I deliberately ignored the fact that it had the opposite effect.

That night, at home, in bed around 3 AM at night, I stared up at the ceiling, feeling totally exhausted, frustrated and unfulfilled. Tears started to flow down my cheeks, softly, slowly, silently. "I cannot keep going this way," I thought. "I seriously need to change, but I have no clue *how*. I've tried so many times before, but it's like I'm destined to not make it. I'm a lost cause."

The next morning, I QUIT SUGAR! For good! I found the magic pill...

That would have been a great success story, wouldn't it? Only it wasn't. Did I stop? Hell no, I did not! Of course not. I didn't put my own needs first, and more importantly, I didn't understand them either. I carried on being exhausted, moody and very sad.

The Universe had a different plan though. It's like it had finally heard my calling and laid some opportunities in front of me, even though a little disguised.

Some weeks later, I came across a video featuring a profound explanation about our relationship with food. I felt drawn to listen to it . The presenter captivated me. He made sense in his approach; it was different from most and it spoke holistically to me. I thought, "Yes! This is great, it can help my partner regain his health! I will have my partner do this; he really needs to get better and stronger, and when he does, we will be 'happy ever after.'"

You see, I was not ready to face MY addiction, so instead I poured my energy into helping my partner improve his health. I was not yet willing to look within myself, so I enrolled my *partner* in the 90-day challenge. I mean, why on earth would *I* jump onto something that was good for ME? I would rather be in the 'comfort' of being the martyr and stay in victimhood a little longer to justify my exhaustion and get some of that all-too-needed attention.

The only flaw to my master plan was facing the harsh reality that my partner did not want to do this. He didn't feel for it, so I was 'forced' to do the program myself. Bummer! In hindsight, I can see this was not a coincidence. The Universe clearly meant the program was to be done by me. The Universe is funny that way.

I fought my way through the program, not really believing in myself and not necessarily happy with everything throughout the 90 days, either — I'll be honest with you about that. I didn't really believe *I* could manage this; it was more for others to do, but at least I could follow along and see what I could learn in order to help my partner.

I got to meet my emotions face to face, I met resistance. I argued heavily with my willpower and rebelled against rules and routines. However, for some strange reason, the process *worked* for me. It struck a chord within me. It's like it spoke to my heart and I felt at home with it. I found the support, understanding and breakthroughs I needed. I discovered a new community to connect with, a tribe of like-minded people. I started feeling good in my own skin again.

I was brave enough to look at my emotional relationship with food and how I had numbed my internal void with sugary sweets, for so many years. I also realized that my stress levels were already so high and my sugar intake spiked it even more. It is as if sugar is to stress what sparks are to flames: fierce and hard to tame.

I broke up with sugar during those 90 days.

We are no longer a thing.

I couldn't believe it, and nor could the people around me.

Slowly but surely, they have not only seen that my new lifestyle remains but I have also planted seeds of hope in them.

I'll be honest with you though, I did bring my ex (sugar) back in for a little while. I needed to test if we were really through with one another. Was I really ready to put myself and my own well-being and energy first, or did I still want the 'comfort' of being in misery and victimhood, of always being tired and unfocused? I am one to rebel a little, to not want to do as others tell me, so of course I needed to test all the theory. Examine myself and how I was feeling.

And then we broke up again.

Now we ARE done.

It just feels so freaking good waking up in the morning feeling energized and ready to take on my day! The beauty of having time and presence to talk and reflect over life with my sons. To look in the mirror and be happy with what I see. To feel that I am the one making decisions in line with me and what

I want... I wouldn't trade that for some quick highs that create havoc in me, and on those around me.

When I have low and challenging periods now — cause hey, life still happens — I know where my sugar drug is if I want it. My FIX is so easily available. It doesn't cost me much to jump back in to my addiction and I don't even have to be a criminal to get it. Yet, if I am brutally honest with myself, it *does* actually cost me A LOT. It costs me my energy, my mood, my focus, my contribution in social life and my time with my kids. I don't fall for it anymore; I cannot.

Do I still eat sweet things, you may ask? Yes, I do.

Humans have a natural craving for sweet things like the natural sweetness in fruits and I love my fruits, in portions. I can even eat treats or desserts, but I am the one choosing how, when, and in which way.

I now drink loads of water every day because it makes me feel good. Now, it is my *vegetables* that I need every day and I feel low if I don't get them. I listen in for what I really want and need in that moment. How funny is that? Even my sons are now looking at their lifestyle, feeling into what makes *them* good and strong, and what is more of a weakening factor for them. At times they stop and check, "could it be an emotional need that should be met, instead of using food?". I take my sons shopping and we choose our greens together, and that did not happen before. They have started trusting in my change and decided to follow my lead slowly but surely. It is truly amazing.

Was I afraid of giving up sugar? Yes I was, very much so.

There was comfort in it; it was a known factor, even if with negative consequences. Being a bit of an epicurean, I was afraid of my food becoming dull, boring and restricted. Now I feel my food is real, alive, varied in taste and really nourishing for me. I don't feel I miss out on anything.

With the return of my energy, my brain fog lifted and my enthusiasm was back — I could start looking again at working on my dreams, my desires and potential projects that I had had in the back of my mind for years. Self-confidence, energy and sparkle were all added bonuses I gladly welcomed!

When I found the key to break up with sugar, I wanted to tell the whole world about it!

Everybody should do the same, I thought, but it doesn't work that way. I came to see from the people closest to me that you only hear what you are ready and open for. You need to be wanting it *yourself* and not for me to want it for you. We are all on different paths and places in life; we have different things we need to face and learn. We can only start making changes when we are ready and willing ourselves, when we know what changes we want, and more importantly *why* we want it.

When I started to listen within to what my REAL need was in the moment of reaching out for the sweets, I became better at making good choices for myself. Maybe what I need is a hug, or someone to talk to, for someone to see me for who I am and give me comfort that I am enough. My need isn't the sweet itself.

You may be taken by surprise when you pay attention to how those 'foods' actually make you feel and your desire to have them may diminish if you focus on filling your *real* needs instead.

This journey touched my life in such a beautiful way and I wanted to give that to others, so I became a coach for this lifestyle, for those who are ready. There is nothing more beautiful than to see the sparkle come alive again in others. In leading me to change my lifestyle, the Universe gave me such a wake up call and I am filled with gratitude for it. When I put my heart into it, I was able to transform my challenges into strengths. When I see others discover their WHY and embrace the same gift, when I see the sparkle in their eyes and their glowing energy and joy, I feel fulfilled deep in my soul. The beauty of seeing the true person come to life again — it is priceless. I feel so grateful for the fact that I never know what spark I may Ignite in others!

What projects and dreams can you set into life when you get back your confidence, your control and your energy? I cannot wait to see what you will bring to the world. And remember — you never know what spark YOU WILL IGNITE when you get going!!

IGNITE ACTION STEPS

First – I ask you to search deeply into WHY you want to break up with sugar. What is your WHY? If you want a change, you've got to do something different. Are you willing to step a little outside of your comfort zone to do what you have never done before?

Water is almost like a magic pill. It is so simple, yet powerful. Very often, when we feel hungry, we are actually thirsty. Gift yourself loads of pure water every day.

Every time you reach out for your go-to food, whether it is cake, candy or chocolate, listen within. Which emotions are you trying to feed, to numb?

We don't need to have all the answers ourselves. Give yourself permission to receive help. Go find your tribe and surround yourself with support from like-minded people and the ones who walk their talk.

Lastly, think about the legacy you are passing on; what role model do you want to be for your closest family and friends, your children? I ask you to lead by example, and plant seeds for others to follow. You never know what spark you may Ignite!

Hilde Jahren - Norway
Mother, WildFit® Coach, Life Coach, Public Speaker and Adventurer
www.coachhilde.com
@Coachhilde

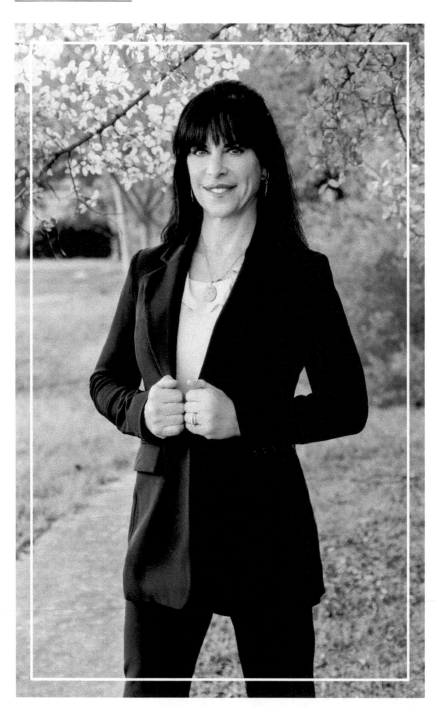

TERESA IRWIN

*"Use your mouth wisely — what goes in, will nourish;
what comes out, will build up others."*

**My goal is to empower women to embrace their femininity and sexuality;
and to also inspire them to take control of their bodies by providing them
with the tools for the prevention of pelvic floor problems and sexual dysfunction. Taking control of her body can help a woman achieve longevity
in the most qualitative way. This has been my journey creating absolute
love and freedom and I share it with you.**

TAKE CONTROL OF YOUR BODY

One of the most deep-seated human needs is the need to feel that we are
in control. As children, one of our first tasks is to learn to control our bodies.
Bladder and bowel function are one of the first areas where we learn to feel
proud of success or shame for failure. We feel that we are 'grown-up' when we
are 'in control.' Of course, this is an illusion because there is so much in life
which we have no control of. Death is the ultimate loss of control.

In my own family, I have seen how facing loss of control can affect someone
severely. When I was 13 years old, my mother, the most amazing and resilient
woman, didn't leave the house for a year! To understand what a huge change
that was, you must understand a little bit about my mother. She grew up in a
remote city in Mexico in a dirt-floored casita without running water. She was
the youngest of 10 (8 survived) and had to quit school in the 6th grade in order

to work and bring home money for family survival. She came to the United States at the age of 18. She was industrious and would buy anything that was extremely "cheap," so that she could turn around and sell it for a profit at swap meets. She ran a maid service, driving the maids to their designated jobs in our old clunky wood-paneled station wagon. My mom even built houses from the ground up (often helping with the manual labor). She did this in the cheapest way possible, determined to make money any way she could, so issues with permits and mechanical problems would sometimes occur.

When I was 13 years old, my youngest brother died at the age of 10. I remember going to the scene where my brother, Keith, was lying in the middle of the highway, with his bicycle laying crushed just a short distance away. Although his face and chest were covered by a policeman's jacket, I recognized my little brother with his cute little non-hairy tanned legs, with sprinkles of blood splattered all around him. My mami (as I would lovingly call her) was behind me, screaming. I can still hear the piercing, murderous-sounding noise she was making, expressing her deepest anguish, as if her life had ended. After that day, she did not leave the house for one full year.

This woman who was able to accomplish so much with drive and ambition could not control everything, and suffered multiple losses throughout her life. My mom lost her first child (a son) at birth; then I was born. Shortly after, my little brother arrived, who was thought to be mentally retarded, later found to be autistic. Then Keith who died in a tragic accident. Her 5th pregnancy ended in a miscarriage. I think that this has made her even more determined to control her remaining children and raise them the way she thought best. It is that battle for control which has defined most of our relationship up until the last several years. There was always something about my decisions that she didn't accept. That left me feeling as if she never saw me, but rather the person she wished I was.

When I became a teenager, naturally trying to gain my independence, my mom had a different plan for me. A deep need to protect me by whatever means she felt was necessary. In the late 1940s and early 1950s, she grew up under a very firm, but NOT controlling mother who was raising eight children of her own in Mexico, of which my mom was the youngest. My mother absorbed my grandmother's life lessons, but in her, they became rigid rules. These strict beliefs, many of which were derived from Catholic beliefs, were carried over and applied to me in their most fundamental and literal way. She protected my ears by not allowing me to know what the word 'pregnancy' meant. She shielded my eyes by not letting me view romantic kissing. She secured my innocence by not permitting me to apply nail polish or wear make-up. She sheltered my heart by secretly listening to my phone calls and reading mail from my boyfriend. She guarded my virginity by shaming sex if performed for any reason other than procreation, and in particular, emphasizing her disgust towards the act of oral sex.

Despite all of that, she encouraged me to be in local beauty and bikini competitions, and placed me in dance performances as well as in cheerleading competitions. She loved making me perform for friends and family, which exhibited the pride she had in me. As a teen, I was lusting for control over my own life, but at the same time, I didn't want to hurt or disappoint her. I loved her and all I wanted to do was make her proud, but the more I tried, the less I felt that was going to happen. I became a hormonally charged screaming teen-ager! I resorted to hiding my actions while trying to achieve independence. I became bulimic, I began to exercise to excess, and took abnormal amounts of laxatives in a quest to be skinny. I did not realize at the time that by doing that, I would prevent normal bowel movements from happening without laxatives. Or that intense stomach cramps would continuously wake me in the middle of the night, making me curl up into a fetal position (and persist in adulthood). I was desperately grasping for control.

In spite of these teenaged behaviors, I did not feel pretty enough, sexy enough, nor did I feel I was deserving enough of praise, although I desperately wanted to hear it from my mom. Her words matter greatly. By needing this, I learned that words can tear you down or build you up. They can persuade you into trying new things you hadn't thought of doing, (possibly negative), or they might also end up becoming positive. It is ultimately how you internalize them.

The communication that we have with anybody and everybody, whether personally or professionally, is critical. It's not just the words, it's the way you present them, and my mother never understood that (at least that is how I felt). Even upon achieving my medical degree as a doctor, she never said she was proud of me. I don't remember her ever telling me that she loved me until I had my own children. Ironically, she told everyone else. It has been a tumultuous journey between us for many years.

In my early twenties, upon reading my mail one day, my mom discovered that I was engaging in pre-marital sex with my fiancé, so she disowned me... I remember this day vividly. My parents had flown into Houston to attend a medical school ceremony celebrating my achievement, but it became an event of shame. My heart was ripped in two. It was the first time I'd experienced such a deep ache in my soul. My poor, sweet dad struggled with my mother's decision to turn her back on me. He would sneak in phone calls, knowing he could get in trouble with her. Because he truly cherished her, while I was the 'apple of his eye,' he never wanted to jeopardize a potential divorce, nor lose communication with me. My daddy is one of the most sincerely tender-hearted people I know.

He has always been by my side, whether it was getting on a scary roller coaster or teaching me how to play baseball in our front yard, or showing me how to drive. He has always been supportive of my decisions, such as going to medical school (instead of raising a family), and even changing my denomination from the one I was raised in. He may not have been happy with some of my actions, but he was forgiving.

My closeness to my father was challenged deeply years later. As a mother of three boys I felt a deep heartbreak when my father took my mother's side in an important family issue. Again, it was a case of my mother exerting control. This was the first time I felt like my father was abandoning me during one of the most important events of my life.

Upon finding out that our teenage son was going to become a father but was not going to get married, my dad became almost belligerent. Interestingly, when he first found out, he was not upset. However, after a few days went by, he began to adopt my mom's sentiments, as she impressed upon him how wrong she felt this was.

I took it so personally, I felt as if I were the one pregnant out of wedlock! This event triggered very painful memories. For so many years, my immediate reaction was to reactively respond in an illogical and negative way to anything I perceived as unsupportive — coming from my mom. It took me many years of conscious work and meditation to logically hear her words and actions and turn them into a positive reaction of acceptance, understanding, and admiration. All that work seemed undone for a while, as the old illogical emotional responses came rushing back. As is usually the case with such things, my daddy as well as my mami eventually came around and I was able to work myself back to a more centered place mentally. Now, they absolutely adore Lily, our granddaughter, as well as her amazing momma!

I have spent years working on forgiveness, understanding my own motivations and thought processes. It was shocking how that could be triggered in just a few minutes. Fortunately though, once that work is done, getting back to that conscious mindset is not as difficult as was getting there initially. Struggles are often the catalysts for growth, and these conflicts with my mother's controlling personality were what started me on the path to focus on understanding WHY she raised me as she did. I remember distinctly when learning the "Laws of Human Nature" by Robert Greene, that I needed to place myself in her shoes.

I began to recall the sacrifice that my mom had made by taking on the full-time job of helping my husband and I take care of our favorite middle son, Tyler, for the first six months of his life. At the time I was still delivering babies as an obstetrician, and often did not come home until after office hours the following day. My mami would bring Tyler and spend the night in the doctor's call room at the hospital so that I could breastfeed him in between deliveries. As I reflected upon this and knowing how intense my love is for our sons, it became as clear as the most beautiful crystal why she raised me in the fashion that she did. It was her way of protecting and maintaining control of the remaining children she had left. Her way of parenting was what she felt was the best for me. She was trying to be my protector — something I did not understand until I became a mother myself.

Knowing that strong love between parent and child helped me see WHY my mami did all the 'protective measures' that she did. I let go of my anger and control I was exerting in my own life, with my own kids. I began doing things that helped me feel in control but in a more constructive and supportive way.

Perhaps it is this long history of struggles for control of my own life that makes me so empathetic to the women in my medical practice. As a urogynecologist (or 'vagina-cologist' as my sons call me) working in female pelvic medicine and reconstructive surgery, I treat pelvic floor dysfunction, such as pelvic organ prolapse, incontinence, pelvic pain, and sexual dysfunction. There is a surprising number of women who have lost control over one of the most basic areas of their lives — control of their own bodily functions. Unfortunately, as women, our bodies undergo changes throughout life over which we often have little control. A large number of women avoid social events, such as the movies, family gatherings, and trips — everyday things the rest of us take for granted — because they are afraid of soiling themselves or having to make frequent awkward visits to the restroom.

There are so many examples of what women have confidentially and embarrassingly told me regarding how their lack of bodily control is affecting their quality of life. One very successful executive, while sitting through a lengthy board meeting, lost control of a large amount of urine! Another patient described how she had to get up every 30 minutes during a movie hauling her grandchildren along with her because of their young ages. This caused a public scene eliciting significant annoyance amongst the movie patrons and her grandchildren. Another woman told me that she avoided sex because she would leak urine with every thrust; while another had complete bladder leakage upon orgasm and still another leaked poop and didn't even realize it until they finished, only to find some feces under her buttocks. My heart aches when I hear these stories of others apologizing, and ashamed, and I sympathize with their situations.

Fortunately, there are multiple treatments I am able to offer these women. I feel so much contentment when I see them return after treatment because I have helped them regain some control back into their lives! How I feel with the gratitude they express, is beyond words...

I have the privilege of using fancy robotic, high-tech instruments to fix pelvic floor problems — problems where the initial damage began in the child-bearing years. I truly love performing surgeries that result in the restoration and improvement in the lives of women affected by those conditions, but it needs to start with **educating** women in their teenage years (and beyond), on the proper and preventative ways to take care of their bodies. By working to maintain and improve the pelvic floor, when a childbirth or other insult occurs, the damage is transient. Women can take control of this!

I see a lot of significant pelvic floor damage in the West, but Africa is far worse. Women who have no access to modern prenatal care can suffer prolonged labors and horrific deliveries with minimal medical assistance. If the baby gets stuck, they usually lose the child, and have such severe pelvic floor damage that they no longer have any bladder and bowel control. They are ostracized and placed in 'fistula clinics,' almost like the historical leper colonies, because no one wants to be around a woman or teenager who is continuously dribbling urine and feces. My dream and hopes are to reduce the number of women in Third World fistula clinics so they can have normal lives. Usually surgery is the only cure — conservative measures will not suffice.

I want to empower women to achieve control through constructive means, contrary to how I initially tried to achieve control through my own self-destruc-tive behaviors. And I want them to do it before the damage begins. Education in prevention must begin early in order to be most effective. I am on a quest to help women regain control of their lives by re-establishing normal bodily functions through behavioral changes. I want them to be able to enjoy all the activities and events that make life so special and rewarding without the fear of losing control. I'm proud of the work I do. And, finally, my mami is able to say how proud she is of me too.

Ignite Action steps

Do your pelvic floor exercises (PFE), previously known as Kegel exer-cises. It's the most critical step that needs to be done for the rest of your life.

The exercise involves repeatedly contracting and relaxing the muscles that form your pelvic floor. It is critical that these exercises be done properly. For PFE to be effective, they need to be performed every day for the rest of your life. It needs to become a habit — can be done while driving, in the subway, in the elevator, wherever and whenever. They are very effective if done, but BIG SURPRISE, they only help if you do them!

Do other exercise too! Some fun forms of exercises that will help strengthen the pelvic floor include yoga, hypopressives, figure 8 fitness, belly dancing, and 'sexercise.' For yoga, poses that target the pelvic floor include happy baby, table top, bridge, goddess, and mermaid; simply add a pelvic contraction to the pose.

Breathe! Hypopressives, or Low Pressure Fitness combines rhythmic breathing patterns with a series of poses and postural exercises. This decreases the internal pressure within your thoracic, abdominal, and pelvic cavities. Traditional core exercises, such as planks and sit-ups are HYPER-pressive, increasing internal pressure. Re-training the involuntary muscle fibers that account for a significant percentage of your core muscle fibers translates to an improvement in the pelvic floor muscles (PFM).

Sexercise! With or without a partner, it is an excellent time to strengthen the PFM. It can also enhance sex for both you and your partner. Performing these exercises during sex increases the vaginal strength, increasing the frictional forces along the length of the vagina. When performed properly, PFE increase blood flow, arousal, and the strength of orgasms.

START EARLY! Many women invariably will have years of minor issues with incontinence, but ignore it until it becomes worse. It does not have to be that way. As Diane Newman, a clinical research DNP and author, states, "Continence is a learned behavior." Behavioral training, as when teaching a child to become 'potty trained,' can also work in adults.

Since PFE are only one of many recommendations for the prevention and/ or treatment of PFD, I recommend that you see a pelvic floor therapist, or a physician, specialized in either Urogynecology, Gynecology, or Female Urology.

Teresa Irwin - United States
MD, FACOG, FPMRS
www.caringcenterforwomen.com
◨ CaringCenterForWomen

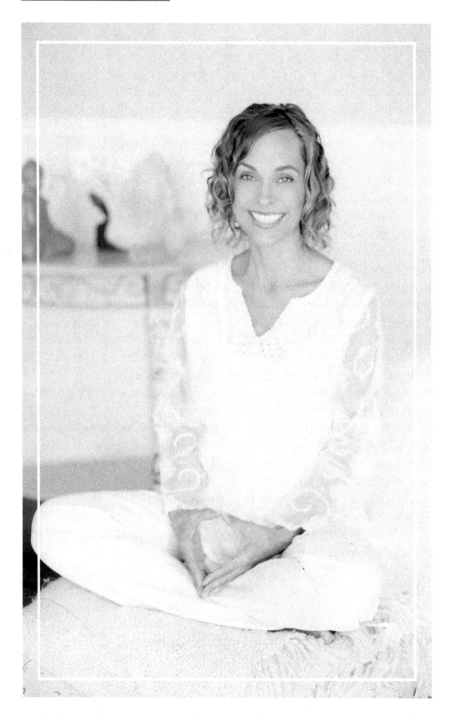

YAANA HAUVROESH

"Choose, in each moment, only the highest vibrational nourishment for your body, mind, heart and soul."

I share my story with you in hopes that you may be inspired to connect more deeply to the healing power of nature, both that which surrounds you and is within you. May you be moved to seek more silence and solitude in the sanctuary of Mother Nature. May you be motivated to explore the healing potential of eating higher vibrational foods and be reminded that your body has an innate wisdom and ability to heal when given the opportunity to do so. May you experience optimal levels of health and wellness!

NOURISHED BY NATURE: INSIDE AND OUT

There I was, alone in the desert, for eleven days and nights with only a small ration of drinking water. And yet, I felt amazing. I was in awe of a connection to self and source that I had not known was possible. Having only water to sustain myself, yet feeling more vital and alive with each passing day, it seemed clear that I was being nourished by something other than food. I was filled with a deep sense of peace, completely trusting in the wisdom of my body and the nature that surrounded me.

It had not always been like that, however. Up until then, my relationship with my body as well as the environment around me had been challenging, to say the least. Neither my own skin nor the world were comfortable for me to inhabit. Growing up I went to school, played with friends, had family dinners, and did my homework just like everyone else. At the same time, I seemed unable to tolerate that which others were at ease with. At school I pleaded with my teachers that my desk be moved away from the chalk dust and the buzz of fluorescent lights. Most mornings, clothes were strewn about my room in a frantic and futile search for something comfortable to wear. Only decades later would I come to understand that it was clean air, full spectrum light and natural fibers that my body was seeking. Needless to say, there were numerous misunderstandings in my growing up years. I appeared challenging and demanding, despite my open-hearted nature and good grades.

By the age of eighteen my body was plagued with digestive complaints, skin rashes, inflammation, and low energy. My mental capacities were diminishing due to brain fog, anxiety, and general malaise. These cognitive symptoms were of great concern given that only a short time before I had graduated at the top of my class. Despite repeated visits to the doctors, no diagnosis or treatment seemed forthcoming. Confused and afraid, the heavy shadows of despair and depression clouded my world — until one day, when I was lent a book which changed everything.

There it was, in black and white. People just like me had simply modified their diet and regained their health. The program called for eliminating sugar, wheat, dairy, yeast, fruits, and fermented foods as well as most of my dietary staples. It appeared that food might in fact be the culprit and source of my ills. That day, I removed almost everything from the refrigerator and cupboards, taking the first steps of what would become a journey spanning three decades. Within the first week, I had regained significant physical vitality, an increase in mental clarity and much greater emotional balance. I was convinced that the foods I had been living on were not only impacting the malfunctioning of my body, but my mind. I was elated to have finally discovered the root of my struggles and the solution. So dramatic was this new lease on life that I continued eating this way for months and years after the recommended six week 'yeast free' protocol, vowing to never again allow food to cause such suffering. I now knew that eliminating certain foods and including others allowed the body to access its own healing potential.

This began my quest for more knowledge on food as medicine. My bible became Paul Pitchford's *Healing with Whole Foods.* I studied macrobiotics at the Kushi Institute, returning home with a deeper understanding of the impact of not only food but also the environment around me. In search of fresh air and clean living, I decided to leave the city and move 'back to the land' with my new husband; enjoying organic gardens, solar power, wood stove, an earth-friendly home, and soon welcoming a baby. As the years passed, I remained committed to living a more simple life, leaving behind the health challenges and confusion of my earlier years. Or so I thought.

When my son turned six years old, I was rushed to the hospital by ambulance with paramedics unable to find a pulse. It was both the most terrifying and transcendent moment of my life. An unforgettable near death experience brought about by an anaphylactic shock left me shattered, both spiritually and mentally. Spiritually, in the best way possible, I was granted access to realms beyond this one. I was graced with an encounter that changed my understanding of who we are and where we come from, eliminating my fear of death or the afterlife. Returning to this earthly plane, however, I was mentally devastated by the implications of what had occurred. I did not understand how it was possible that my body had failed me, how the good living and healthy eating had not protected me. I had almost died, and no one could explain why. There was no known allergen or conclusive test results and therefore no way to ensure that it would not happen again. As my mind grasped for answers, I flashed back to those earlier years when my health had been compromised. At that time, it was only *my* well-being that was at stake. Now things were different. I had someone else to live for and to take care of. My son needed his mother to be alive and healthy. I was determined to make that so.

With this new level of conviction, a much deeper quest commenced. I incorporated the principles of food combining, ayurvedic teachings and traditional Chinese medicine. I became a vegetarian, then vegan, eventually raw foodist, followed by sproutarian and juicarian. Cupboards were filled with the best supplements and superfoods available. Determined to leave no stone unturned, my search for answers extended to consultations with practitioners of acupuncture, naturopathy, homeopathy and more. I travelled to various centers such as Hippocrates and The Ann Wigmore Institute to learn from those leading the way in using food as medicine.

I also sought out ways to quiet my mind and balance my emotions through meditation, yoga, chi-gong, mindfulness training and personal growth seminars. The body/mind connection captivated me; I wanted to learn more about the workings of the human psyche and its influence on the body's ability to heal. All of this led me to pursue postgraduate studies in body-centered psychotherapy and become a licenced counselor offering my clients this integrated and holistic approach to their healing.

What showed up next on my journey was unexpected. I was invited to participate in a Vision Quest. I thought to myself that as much as I wanted to experience a vision and have clarity on my next steps, I was not so sure about being out in the middle of the desert alone. I had never spent much time hiking or camping in the wild, and certainly not on my own. I did not know how to start a fire with twigs alone, or find my way in the dark by the guidance of the North Star. And yet, something was calling me to go. With both trepidation and anticipation, I decided to say yes. Immediately after doing so, I wondered what I had done. Not only was I going to be without human contact, but also without food, the very thing which kept me healthy and well. As the days got closer, I questioned my decision. Food was such an integral part of my world; I needed it for optimal functioning. And what if my body went into another reaction, indeed there would be no paramedics or ambulance nearby. I would be out in nature without anyone or anything to assist me. I asked myself if I was really going to go through with this?

And, apparently I was. A few weeks later, with just my sleeping bag and water, I set out from the base camp and wandered through the desert in search of my sacred space to sit in solitude. Just as the sun was beginning to set, I finally found that perfect bluff of sand overlooking the ocean, where I would be alone for the next eleven days.

Or so I thought.

That first night, I learned how inhabited the desert actually is. I was visited by sand crabs tugging on my sleeping bag, serenaded by the chirping of crickets and kept company all night long by an infinite number of stars above. As the days went by, I came to discover that I was also surrounded by that which I could not detect with my five senses, that which was beyond the world of form. I started to feel the life force that was pulsating around me in the vast emptiness created by sand and sea. The more that I connected and communed with this energy, the more vitality and aliveness I experienced within myself. Although I had set out on this journey wondering how my body was going to survive without food, I realized that with each breath I was being nourished by the elements that surrounded me. And, I had never felt better!

It was an epiphany as they say, a realization that changed me forever. There I was, without food, and yet experiencing the furthest reaches I had ever known of physical vitality, mental clarity, emotional balance and spiritual connection. I was freed from the bondage that food had held over me for so many decades. At last, I was liberated by expanding my understanding of what constituted 'nourishment.'

I was feasting on breakfasts of the most incredible kaleidoscope of colors as the sun rose each day and shone its morning light on a fresh canvas. My dinner was a palette of equally exquisite colors that were painted every evening by the rays of the setting sun.

Throughout the days I dined upon the sights, sounds and smells of all that surrounded me. I was nourished by the songs of the birds, the touch of the breeze, the fragrance of cactus and the ocean air, as well as the warmth of the sand embracing me as I lay back and gazed up at the clouds floating above. Almost every moment there was something for the senses to devour and delight in. I had no idea that being alone in silence and solitude, with nothing, could taste so good and be so completely intoxicating!

This rich buffet of endless options offered new surprises every day. One afternoon while sitting in meditation and asking to be shown my next steps, I opened my eyes to see the most incredible display of power and playfulness bursting up from the surface of the ocean in front of me. There were dozens of manta rays lifting themselves up and out of the water, soaring many feet into the air and then gracefully turning to fall again beneath the surface of the water. There was a symphony of rhythmical sound and vibration, as one after another, these majestic sea creatures crashed down upon the waves. I would have thought it not possible unless I had seen with my own eyes, this incredible feat of defying both the weight of water and gravity to create such a dance of celebration. As I sat captivated by this performance, I was overwhelmed by wonder and awe. Tears of absolute joy and delight ran down my cheeks as spontaneous laughter emerged.

My heart was filled with gratitude for this display of joyful liberation from perceived limitations. This was the answer to my question: *liberation from limitations*! It was such a visually stunning demonstration of the magic possible when we reach further and higher, when we break free from our perceived constraints. This message was delivered so eloquently, with such joy and playfulness, that I raised my head and whispered "thank you" over and over to the heavens. I couldn't imagine anything more delicious or healing! It was better than any organic gourmet meal! It was an Ignite moment indeed!

When the eleven days ended, I wasn't ready to leave my sanctuary or return to physical food. I was the last of the group to arrive at basecamp, and unlike the other questers who enjoyed a feast that evening, I continued for another ten days living on coconut water and green juices. These twenty-one days set me upon a new exploration and became the first of many extended fasts. In awe of what was possible when the body was given the opportunity to access its own healing capacities, I traveled to Hawaii for water fasting with Dr. Cassar and to the Dead Sea for a spiritual fast with Dr. Gabriel Cousens. The results were inspiring and brought further inquiry.

290 / Yaana Hauvroesh

I started to wonder how my life might have been different had I known about fasting decades ago. I questioned everything that I had studied prior to this discovery, and asked myself if any of it had been necessary. I wondered if all of the time, money and energy that had been invested in foods, products, treatments and programs could have been avoided through the use of fasting. Upon reflection however, I came to see that each step along the way had been an essential part of my healing journey. I realized it had been a process and progression up the spiral of conscious and 'evolutionary eating.' This soon formed the basis of a program I shared with others, supporting a gradual transition from foods that were more dense and solid, to choices that were lighter and had a higher frequency. Wherever they were at, we worked together to move them incrementally and step by step closer to 'high vibrational nourishment' — a phrase I used to encompass all the elements we are fed by: air and water, music and aromas, landscape and sunshine, as well as the people and thoughts we surround ourselves with.

All of this led naturally to my next quest of finding remote places where I could take those who were interested in a deeper understanding of the healing power of nature and their own body's wisdom. Providing an experience of being immersed in the elements but still with some creature comforts and conveniences became a new passion and pursuit. It is a joy and a delight to encourage those who may not otherwise journey into the wild, to push beyond their limits and experience a deeper connection to self and source than they may have known previously.

Inviting you, the reader, to find your own way to immerse yourself in nature and deepen your connection to the earth elements while allowing your body to access its own healing potential. Reminding you that by choosing higher vibrational nourishment on all levels, food and beyond, you will be guided and supported to actualize your highest potential—body, mind, heart, and soul.

Ignite Action Steps

Connect to the healing elements of mother nature:
AIR............. Breathe fresh clean air and oxygen deeply into your lungs.
SUN........... Receive the warmth of the sun's rays upon your skin and eyes.
EARTH...... Walk (barefoot if possible), sit and lay down upon the earth.
WATER...... Be near, touch and immerse yourself in fresh and saltwater.
ETHER....... Sense the energy and aliveness in the empty space around you.
HEAVENS... Make time for stargazing and sleeping outside under the moon.

Ask yourself this question: "How can I commit to more fully and consistently taking in the gifts of nature on a regular basis?" And how can I follow through?

Take out your calendar and schedule to spend time in nature. Plan to have some bite size nourishment daily, indulge in a full day each month and allow for a deeper connection at least one weekend each quarter.

1. **Choose high vibrational nourishment:** Support your own wisdom and healing power with 'high vibrational nourishment' for your body, mind, heart, and soul. *Ask yourself " How can I...*
   - *sleep more in harmony with the natural rhythms of the earth?*
   - *improve the quality and source of my drinking water?*
   - *increase my intake of organic, local and plant-based foods?*
   - *learn more about and experiment with daily intermittent fasting?*
   - *use more natural fibers and products on my body and in my home?*
   - *choose exercise and movement that brings me more joy?*
   - *find ways to reduce my exposure to WiFi and electronic devices?*
   - *surround myself with more of the colors and objects that I enjoy?*
   - *play music and sounds that bring me more joy and upliftment?*
   - *bring more elevating aromas into my home and workplace?*
   - *connect with more people who nurture and enrich my life?*
   - *be more mindful of choosing thoughts that support my desires?*
   - *create more solitude and silence for deeper connection with self?*

2. **Consider a deeper immersion:** Research the different programs that offer vision quests or fasting and schedule your own experience! Or perhaps start with programs that provide a deeper experience of high vibrational living through both food and natural surroundings. Allow yourself to be supported and guided in the process of immersing into the healing power of nature and your body's own wisdom.

Yaana Hauvroesh MA., RPC. - Canada
Body-Centered Psychotherapist, Marriage & Family Counselor,
High Vibrational Lifestyle Consultant
info@purestessence.com
www.purestessence.com

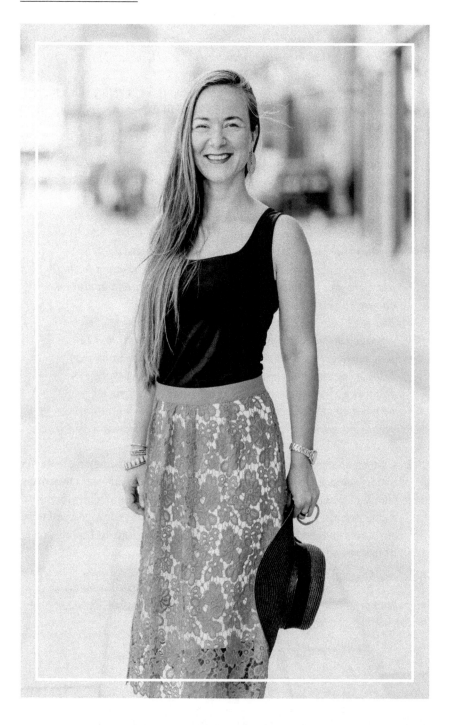

Inga Ulmane

"The body is a tool for reaching higher than you ever thought; both a reflection and a messenger for limitless living."

My purpose is to inspire people that we all are able to live and experience limitless lives. Our physical bodies and physical capacity are not the ones setting boundaries to our dreams or ambitions. Our bodies are here to help us to fulfill our wishes, goals and desires; they are our partners, so long as we don't abandon them but cooperate and respect them!

Limitless Life

As long as I can remember, I have always had long hair down to my tailbone. As a teenager, I loved having long hair. I loved receiving compliments for my hair. I never complained about how long it took to wash and dry it as I was so proud of it. As a teen, I was very involved in school activities, non-governmental movements, in charity work, and other pursuits. I ran from one activity to the next, always hurrying, always trying to fit more into my day, but I always managed to find time for my hair, even when it was an obstacle to getting enough sleep.

Many years later, I found myself standing next to the bathtub, my head bowed down so I could wash my hair without getting the rest of my body wet. If someone were filming me, most probably it would look like I had a super itchy scalp — I was massaging with very anxious and rapid movements (rather like scratching in a panic) the shampoo in my hair. It was like my life would depend on how fast I could wash my hair, or maybe someone was counting the seconds I took to clean it and the million dollar prize would be awarded to the fastest one. In reality — I was at my parent's home. They were looking after my two-year-old son and finally I had time to close the bathroom doors behind me to enjoy some 'me' time undisturbed by my child, work, or someone calling. Taking this time was a luxury.

I had a habit of being super busy. Work, family, everything needed a lot of my attention. Finding time for myself was rare, and all the more so now since my beloved husband had just passed away six months before. Since his passing, I had been keeping the same speed in my social, professional, family, charity and physical activities. Actually, I had been speeding them up rapidly since his death. I promised him I would not grieve, but I would live the dreams and values we both believed in. I made a promise to myself too — I will prove that as a single mom, I can still live a fulfilled, self-realizing life. His death doesn't mean I have to give up on my dreams and ambitions — ambitions that have never been small.

I was 27 years old at that moment at my parents. I had a moment of realization remembering how during all my teenage years, I had been wondering about the mental and physical capacity of a human being — how far can we go without losing a life or a mind? What is the limit, and is there actually a limit? I researched case studies, followed by mental health campaigns, watched documentaries, read research papers... and more.

It was a sudden moment of guilt, of being aware and conscious of my status quo. I was looking at myself from afar and I lost hope for a moment, thinking that my life and situation had proven what I feared the most — that there *were* limits to a human's capabilities. Obviously I was not ready to accept it nor to change my belief of limitless life. I was wondering how long I was going to keep it up.

I had already experienced three burnouts at the time, five types of gastritis, and had a duodenal ulcer. My memory had grown shorter than that of a goldfish. I had trembling fingers, iron, vital vitamin and mineral deficiencies. I was developing autoimmune and hormonal imbalances, and thyroid issues. Most probably the list could have been at least twice as long if I wouldn't have been so immune toward prioritizing myself and neglecting the Western healthcare and medicine.

One would think—God willing, she would open her eyes and stop chasing the dreams at the speed of light, but instead take care of herself.

My friends and family respected me for my way of getting over my husband's death, but they kept on worrying. I didn't slow down and the opposite happened. I *needed* extra pressure... or so I thought. So, I decided to move to the Middle East, away from Latvia, the most amazing natural and peaceful country I have ever known, and where I had all the support system I needed: my parents, friends and colleagues. I left everything: my friends, family, social and charity activities, my whole mental and emotional support system. I was a single mom with a kid and a high status job position with impressive official titles that required my attention 24/7. There was no financial support and I had no intentions of looking for a nanny or any household help. Despite my impressive and significant job position, time restraints and getting adjusted to the new country and environment, I felt I had to give my son the love of two — so he did not feel the shortage of one of the parents and the love and security he needed. I knew that if I had the additional help of a nanny I would become a miserable workaholic.

The sudden awareness during that hair washing moment was way too short. My stubborn high achiever's mind needed a harder and longer awakening. And it came. Thanks to my hair. Again. I always used to say I might not have the body of a model, but my hair is my long-lasting treasure and that awareness kicked me painfully. I started losing my hair! It didn't happen all at once, but it was definitely noticeable. With hair as long as mine, when even a few long hairs fall out, it looks like a lot more as it curls and tangles in the bottom of the tub. It looks like at least a dozen hairs have fallen out. Imagine when numerous strands of hair fall out during a single wash. Seeing my hair lying there gave me a panic attack! My long-time identity, my treasure and my 'curtain to hide behind' was falling out at high speed!

The hair loss continued over the next half a year in an accelerated rhythm. I was blessed with kind of thick hair so you couldn't see it right away and the length of the hair did not make it so obvious, but for me, this trivial signal was it! I just knew that I had to make big changes in my life, and I had to do it fast. While living in a desert concrete jungle I managed to take a breath and promised myself I would research, test and try every little thing to reverse this... and I would take it to the next level.

And of course—it could not involve any doctors because I could and I had to solve it MYSELF. Because I COULD. So I had to become 'a doctor', my own doctor and my own support mechanism as I had no one except a very demanding career, the challenging environment of the Middle East, and my amazing son (but I did not want to put any responsibility or load on him).

From there, I started a practical way of becoming a doctor — I became a biohacker. I started hacking the secrets of physical and mental experience, my insistent passion for limitless life. I believed there was a way for me to manage it all and even more — without health consequences, and so I found biohacking.

My definition of biohacking is finding the convenient and sustainable ways of raising a human being's performance without compensating, questioning or harming one's health. It is like a box of tools you can improvise with when you need to, when ambition grows and the higher goal is there, or when the life offers some new challenges or obstacles. And so, prompted by the condition of my health, I started experimenting.

I had been vegan for some period of time, then a raw eater, then I did not eat at all for days and fasted. When the new research and case studies came out, I became a total meat lover, got quite constipated for a long time, ran for 15 kilometers every day, gained kilograms, lost eight kilograms in four weeks, and so on. The list of experiments grew so long that I could write a book about it. In trying so many methods, in experimenting with my own self, I kept on working the wrong way—causing and then fighting the consequences, as today's healthcare system does and promotes doing — keep on hiding the dust under the bed and hope the monster does not wake up and scare you one fine day.

The more I read, the more it got me thinking. In the middle of 20th century, all the automotive industry was developing cars with a mindset of 'solving the consequences of accidents' — building a more durable frame of the car so the human body gets less affected during the damage caused by an accident, creating airbags, relocating the location of the engine, pulling the steering wheel back from the driver, etc. The automotive industry was brainstorming how to make any car a safer place for a human's body during an accident. It wasn't until the idea to control the moment right before the accident came in the mid 1990s when an increasing amount of data from real-world accidents began being incorporated into development efforts that the industry started to develop more efficient brakes, introduce new driving laws like keeping distance between the cars, improving the seatbelts, and so on.

Nowadays, this evolution has grown to companies working on driverless cars (which claim to be way safer than a human-led vehicle), on steering wheels that function as heart rate monitors for drivers with risk factors for heart attack — always evolving in an attempt to avoid any possible car crash and potential accidents on the streets.

This helped me to draw parallels to the convenient healthcare system we use today all over the world. We notice concerns then we wait for the worst to happen. It's hard to diagnose things accurately and often, we resort to a method of exclusion. We try treatments for symptoms and then, if they work, announce that must have been the correct diagnosis, regardless of the truth of it.

As Justin Timberlake sings, "the damage is done so I guess I be leaving..." — a diagnosis is made, a solution prescribed, and regardless of potential short term and long term consequences, the medical system believes its job is complete with no more to be done. But what if we could flip it and focus our efforts on preventive healthcare?

This is where the game began for me. I started reading every book I could find on health, nutrition, food as medicine, and mindset around it until it became my purpose: not only to guide myself towards a higher quality of life but also to help others. Friends started to come to me for advice. They trusted my nutritional advice and food plans, but I wanted to play the real game, so I started studying health and nutrition on a bigger scale. Digging deep, I took it to the next level.

Every day, I worked to deepen my understanding of 'biohacking' because I continue to choose the limitless life. I started working primarily with two different modalities. I became a certified PRECISION NUTRITION Level 1 Nutrition coach and also a facilitator of PSYCH-K®. These two different modalities, one physical and the other mental, helped me define a framework for what I was trying to do. One is focused on a surface level, working with the body physically on a tangible level. The other examines how you program your body and mind mentally, consciously and subconsciously. I believe a limitless life can be reached by combining and mastering the physical, mental and spiritual worlds in a conscious and mindful way.

This summer my good friend dared me to cut my hair to step into my womanhood and change my overall image. Instead, I respected the loyalty I felt to my long-term partner — the hair that has always been there in good and bad times, the loving companion who opened my eyes and showed me to be aware of my health and it was time to change.

I sometimes feel as if I have put a new pressure on myself again — in regards to the new part of the world I am living in. I have chosen to develop one more career— biohacking, while living already full of titles and responsibilities. My son is also growing up and he takes a lot of my energy to spend quality time with him. I am forever reading parenting books on how to do it the best possible way. I have always loved my own approach to keep me motivated, that I call — move 'your ass and your mind will follow.' I have learned to listen to my body and its issues. I approach it as a wise messenger — giving me signals when I am taking the best appropriate and beneficial path for me or vice versa. Now I have become grateful to any pain, to any uncomfortable feeling in my body because it serves as a signal to listen and reflect on. I am always one breathwork, one meditation, one week in a fasted state away from resetting my body or mental state. And it feels amazing! It is like dancing with a partner: sometimes you have to grab his hand and sometimes you have to let him grab yours. I have learned to use these tools to increase my energy, but also to increase my productivity so I can spend less time and get better results at work, while sleeping and eating appropriately so my memory and mind is sharp and ready to accept the new knowledge I need. The most important thing I have learned is — to say NO to others and myself, when I am getting too busy to listen to my body and putting recovery as a priority.

Trust your body. It is your greatest companion. The body is a tool to help reach the highest version of you. It is both a reflection and a messenger for limitless living.

Are you ready for a limitless life full of amazing health and energy?

IGNITE ACTION STEPS

1. Measure anything and everything about your body; information is one of the most powerful tools.

What gets measured gets achieved. Human bodies are like complex, spacious and very generous data machines — anything can be measured, observed and analyzed. And any data or information is the tool you need to get one step closer to success. When it comes to health nowadays, simple blood panels can be done. You can analyze your DNA and potential related risks, sleep patterns, your ability to meditate and focus, the body's response to certain diets, products, work loads, routine or exercises. Basically anything, including your biological age can be identified. It doesn't have to be an expensive test in a lab—even observing oneself after eating different foods, exercises and sleep routines. You can create some conclusions on what is more beneficial for your health, body, mind and mood. If you listen closely enough the body tells you everything you need to hear.

2. Your body and health condition (emotional and physical feeling) is the wisest messenger of all.

Whenever you have a health issue, even a stiff back, pain in your shoulder, or your back bothers you—question it—what does the pain want to tell you?

What do you get from treating it? Attention? Self love? Time for yourself? Nurturing? Those are quite often the answers.

Once you begin listening to your body and have given what it needs, the pain magically releases or disappears. Nowadays the 'quick fix' medicine approach is actually helping us to shutdown a powerful information channel — our own bodies. Once you numb and silence it, you lose a connection (like with the radio). The more you ignore it, the louder and more noticeable the pain (or disease) will come out and scream for attention.

3. Develop critical thinking when it comes to doctors, diagnosis and healing your condition.

Don't follow trendy campaigns, influencers, opinion leaders or 'over-opinionated' movies calling themselves documentaries. In our society, in this century, we are lacking critical thinking. While professionals in the healthcare system may lack an open mind and not always take time to listen closely to the patient, we need to develop healthy, critical thinking towards statements regarding our well being. When you have an issue, read about it, question yourself when you got it, why you might have attracted it and don't be afraid to do some research. I am not saying to listen to the Dr. 'Google' about everything, but medicine and healthcare is evolving so fast that you might find some new research that your doctor may not be aware of.

4. Don't be afraid to experiment.

I want to remind you of my own philosophy that I am living by — 'Move your ass and your mind will follow.' Be open-minded to new alternatives. Challenge traditional methods along with your old limitations and habitual thinking. Break free from beliefs you have created from the past. Try different natural, body-friendly and sustainable methods. Cold exposure, intermittent fasting and breathwork are great things to begin with. Listen to how your body responds to these new experiences and give it time.

Inga Ulmane - Latvia and United Arab Emirates
Biohacker, Nutrition and lifestyle coach, Psych-K® facilitator
inga.ulmane@gmail.com
www.ingaulmane.com

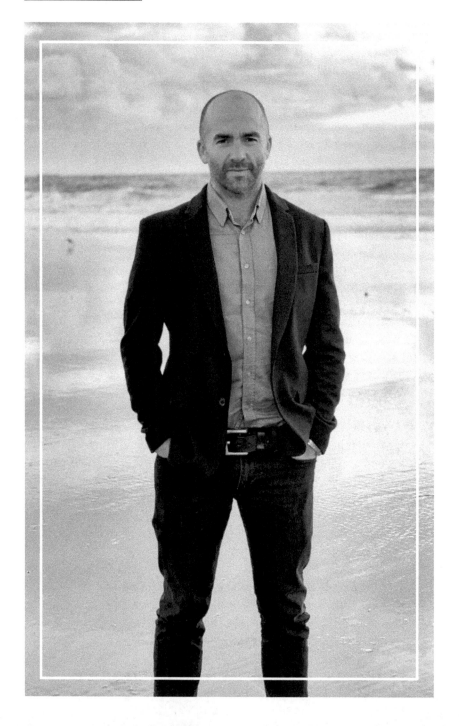

NEIL CANNON

*"Your body's ability to heal is greater than you
have ever been allowed to believe."*

**My desire is to remind you of how beautifully intelligent and powerful
the human body is at healing itself. When you read my story, I want you
to be filled with new knowledge and inspiration, and to know that when
you address the root cause of your symptoms, you can ignite your inner
healer, free yourself from any illness, pain and medication and live a life
rich in vitality.**

IGNITE YOUR INNER HEALER

I've come to understand that everyone who works in holistic health has their
own story of healing or knows of someone who has healed something beyond
the comprehension and limits of Western medicine. I expect you can relate to
this if you've ever seen a holistic practitioner.

For as long as I can remember, until recent years, I suffered from constant
eczema. When I was very young, I would be always scratching my skin. My
red and raw skin and scabs would get strange looks. I'd go to bed wearing
white gloves to ensure I wouldn't scratch. Quite often, I'd wake up with holes
in the fingers of bloody gloves.

In school, I'd occasionally get teased, not a great deal, but enough for it to
matter. I wouldn't say I was bullied, but I was a little self-conscious, particularly
as no one else in my class appeared to suffer from it. I was the one with eczema.

It almost became part of my identity. It was mainly on my hands, wrists, inside of my elbows and behind my knees. In the winter it would crack open and in the summer it would itch and weep.

I remember hearing that people would grow out of it — this didn't happen with me. As I entered secondary school, it seemed to get progressively worse. In times of stress, particularly around the time of my exams, it spread onto my neck, arms and back. In my teens, it seemed to be everywhere. I'd regularly go to the doctor to fetch the usual: steroid creams, moisturizers and antibiotics when it got infected. The eczema would heal, then return. These treatments were short-term solutions. Little did I know that this very approach to treat eczema caused more harm than good and it ignored entirely why it was there in the first place.

I'll never forget a particular occasion, in my mid-teens, when I sat opposite my doctor after I had experienced a nasty eczema flare up. He examined me. He then went back to his desk and looked at his computer screen. He then looked at me over the screen and asked, "Are you allergic to penicillin?"

"I don't think so," I replied.

As he typed up the prescription for antibiotics, he asked, "Would you like more steroid cream?"

"Yes please," I politely replied. He reminded me to use it sparingly as he glanced at me, before turning back to his screen. I was perplexed. I remember thinking to myself, "Is he just cross-referencing my eczema with drug options?" I remember experiencing this feeling of… helplessness. Not just helpless, but almost cheated. I was expecting something more. Something useful or at least different. I left with the usual prescription and walked to the pharmacy, thinking, "Something is not adding up here."

Little did I know that about 20 years later I'd uncover not only the underlying cause of my eczema and how to reverse it very quickly, but also the root cause of why my doctor kept on prescribing the same treatments visit after visit. I later learned these treatments were only *masking* the symptoms. They did not address why my eczema was there in the first place. In other words, I uncovered the truth about the training provided to conventionally-trained medical professionals. Reflecting now, I feel that my passion for wellness, vitality and healing (and later my career) began in my mid-teens during that moment of perplexity in the doctor's office.

I was told the steroid creams weren't good to use frequently and, as I got older, I felt less inclined to use them. Even with that knowledge, it didn't stop me from relying on them again in my early twenties at university when it flared up again. After graduation, I took some time to myself, to avoid the corporate world for as long as I could. I wasn't ready to spend my life working in an office just yet. My friends from university were all getting real jobs. That wasn't for me! Instead, I worked a winter season as a snowboarding resort rep, traveled and lived in the sunny east coast of Australia, and worked on the stunning island of Corsica as a windsurf instructor. In Corsica, when I wasn't teaching, I'd often be on rescue boat duty. I'd sit on the hot rubber sides of the rescue boat by myself, in the middle of a huge bay, looking out over the waves and daydreaming.

My skin was perfect and I was in the best shape of my life. The sun and sea were a miracle cure and I was active all day long. Just as nature intended. I'd often ponder what I could do with my life, and a couple of things would come to mind. *If I could find a cure for eczema, I'd become a very successful man.* I used to be very money-oriented back then. Now, my goal is to inspire people to be empowered around their health, so they can heal themselves and stop suffering unnecessarily. Perhaps my daydreaming back then was planting the seeds of my future discoveries.

After years of avoiding 'real' work, I reluctantly decided to go back to university and study a Masters in Real Estate Investment. I always had a passion for property development. Low and behold, the eczema returned with a vengeance during the stress of study and pressure. I'd have flare ups throughout my late twenties and during my various jobs in the corporate world in London. I'll never forget walking into the office one day after a night out and a friend of mine exclaimed, "Whoa!! What's happened to your face?!" I had scratched my forehead to pieces. She was laughing, and so was I as I sheepishly attempted to hide my face from her. I sat down at my desk and noticed a few strange looks from my colleagues. I didn't let on to the others, but I felt embarrassed, and laughed it off in an effort to dismiss it.

After being made redundant from that job, I moved away from the corporate world. I spent a few years doing interior renovations. Already passionate about health and fitness, and with a desire to earn a living online to support my love of travel, I decided to write an ebook. My book idea was a combination of my desire to get into online marketing and to solve a specific problem for which hundreds of thousands of men were seeking a solution. It was titled *The Truth About Man Boobs*. I discovered some extraordinary information about how men's hormones, namely testosterone levels, sperm counts and chest area were being affected by all kinds of environmental estrogens. It kickstarted a newfound passion in wellness and healing.

In 2014 I moved to Los Angeles. It was suggested to me that I broaden my market, even though the specific subject matter was of great importance and value. I rebranded to *Mojo Multiplier: Raise Testosterone Naturally*. Around the same time, my father sadly suffered a stroke. It shook him and the family. I'll never forget him telling me in the kitchen of our family home, a few years prior to his stroke, that his doctor had diagnosed him with chronic inflammation. I wasn't really sure what that was. I just knew it sounded like bad news. Shortly after his stroke, I got curious as I kept on seeing this word 'inflammation' in my research. One particular article in a health magazine that my sister had given me was entitled: "What Lies Beneath: It Could Be The Most Important Health Problem You've Never Heard About." It was about inflammation. This really got the ball rolling. I was convinced my father's stroke was avoidable. I had an inner knowing. My heart was telling me something.

It initiated a rabbit hole investigation which was larger than I'd ever imagined. Not only did I discover this underlying cause was entirely reversible naturally — and only naturally — but also that his doctor hadn't made any of the recommendations I'd come across. Chronic or systemic inflammation is not treatable with a drug. It requires getting to the inflammatory root cause and addressing it. Sadly, my father was prescribed medications that masked the root cause, allowing it to worsen unnoticed.

I've found that this is true for the vast majority of medications on the market. Every drug bar none comes with side effects and many will create side effects for which another drug is prescribed; hence the 'pill for a pill' society in which we live. It is almost a social 'norm' to be on a cocktail of medications. I've come to realize that this is not a biological norm. The human body is not that poorly designed that it requires synthetic drugs to keep it thriving. We do not get sick because of a pharmaceutical drug deficiency.

My first 'aha moment' was the discovery that every common and chronic illness and accelerated biological aging is a result of one underlying cause: chronic inflammation. It didn't take me long to find out how to reverse chronic inflammation, and I decided to change a few things about my life — diet and behavioral patterns. In weeks, my eczema disappeared. I must be clear, I can't say it's 'cured.' If I don't follow my own advice, it can come back. Eczema is a symptom of inflammation. Just like any other inflammatory condition, the names given to any 'illness' or a 'dis-ease' are almost irrelevant. I prefer to just call them 'symptoms of X.' Symptoms are messengers, like warning lights in the car, indicating change is necessary in some form.

Throughout the last four years, I've realized that similar principles can be applied to so many health challenges, achieving extraordinary results. I've helped people reverse a myriad of symptoms or 'illnesses' like type-2 diabetes, arthritis and even Parkinson's with similar approaches.

You might be wondering about genetics tendencies or predisposition? In the science of epigenetics, it is now known that it's the environment in the body that signals our genes, and thus the health of our cells and body. In other words, our genes have very little role to play in whether or not we develop an illness. The environment in the body is what triggers illness or wellness. This is true for at least 95 percent of the population. Less than 5 percent of illnesses are a result of genes that are 'fully penetrant,' which means people in that proportion might be born with a 'defective' gene. For the 95 percent majority, we have an immense amount of power to avoid — and heal — our symptoms.

I found that truly empowering to know. What impacts our internal environment? Simply put: what we're putting in our bodies, how physically active we are, sunlight, sleep, what we're exposed to in our external environment, toxins like heavy metals (mercury), fungi, parasites, infections, and how well we're managing our thoughts and emotions. And on a higher level, it's our perception of our world around us that impacts our biology. Our thoughts and emotions can make us sick. And they can make us well.

My initial focus and passion was in nutrition and healing the gut, and it ventured far deeper into the mind-body connection. Whilst nutrition is imperative to get right if you're experiencing any kind of chronic symptom, dealing with nutrition alone is not always going to get results. Some will switch to an anti-inflammatory diet and get results. Others will need to go deeper.

One of my main focuses is skin health, which is so closely tied to gut health. On the subject of the gut, I was recently approached by a newly medically qualified doctor in Sydney, Australia. She told me she was covered in head-to-toe dermatitis. Following her training, she used steroids, antibiotics, and immunosuppressants... and ended up in the hospital. Looking beyond her training, she found me on YouTube. I asked her what she'd learned about gut health and skin health during her training. She said, "Nothing."

Instead, she told me her dermatologist had categorically told her there is no relationship between gut health and skin health. I told her that's the equivalent of being told that there is no relationship between the engine in your car and your car moving. When you heal the gut, you can heal the body and alleviate so many symptoms. Not knowing this can create a lot of unnecessary suffering.

Our emotions play a huge role in a balanced gut. And with my eczema, I knew this only too well. My stress levels and nerves impacted my gut. My chronic stress could make me sick. And my eczema could also become pleasurable (from scratching that itch), addictive, habitual and unconscious.

The other side of that emotional equation is how trapped emotions impact our electrical body. We truly are electrical beings. Trapped emotions are electromagnetic bundles of energy which are stored throughout the body. This trapped energy compromises the flow of electricity through our electrical systems. Our organs are all wired on different circuits, much like a power circuit in the house, and trapped emotions can block the flow of electricity across these systems, as can mercury in the mouth, root canals and cavities. You can release these trapped emotions using a number of different approaches, such as trauma release exercises, yoga and acupuncture.

My second 'aha moment' in my seven-year career in health, wellness and healing, took place when I started exploring the history of the medical system and the role of capitalism through the introduction of patented petrochemicals. By the early 20th century, business moguls led the world of medicine away from natural methods of healing (medicine) and put into place an education system taught to doctors which was heavily biased towards prescription drug therapy (medication). This is why conventionally trained medical professionals today know little to nothing about nutrition or healing. In essence, they created a disease and symptoms maintenance system and a recurring revenue business model. I believe knowing this truth results in a truly empowered state. It's one in which we can rediscover just how powerful the human body is in healing *itself*. One of my favorite quotes is by a creature named Yoda. He said, "You must unlearn what you have learned."

For me the exciting part of this is understanding the sheer power of the mind-body connection and our ability to heal through thought alone. This is an area that thrills me so much right now, and with the latest discoveries of quantum physics, people are achieving what we'd previously describe as only *miracles*. 'Incurable' and supposed 'terminal' diseases are being completely reversed. We are more powerful than we've ever been allowed to believe.

I encourage you so strongly to become your own personal best health advocate — to become your own best doctor and to step outside of the mainstream way of doing things. Every one of us can step into our own true power to heal ourselves when we choose to. When you address the physical, mental, emotional and spiritual pillars of Vitality, you can reach the root cause of any symptom and Ignite your inner healer.

IGNITE ACTION STEPS

You can free yourself from common, chronic illness, pain and repeated use of medications. Address the Physical (nutrition, movement, lifestyle), Mental (thoughts and beliefs), Emotional (feelings and emotions) and Spiritual 'Pillars of Vitality' in the following ways:

1. Remember that your body is an immensely powerful, immaculately designed, self-healing machine. No one gets sick from a pharmaceutical deficiency.

2. Ensure you are getting sufficient oxygen flowing around your body, and that you are physically active. "Sitting is the new smoking." You can't outsource movement and oxygen is our #1 cell and life fuel. Move, daily, a lot. Consider yoga or dance. Pick movement that you enjoy.

3. Drink the cleanest and purest water money can buy. Research your local water supply, invest in filtration, ionization and structured water. Water is our #2 cell and life fuel.

4. Switch to an anti-inflammatory diet, one which suits you. "Let thy food be thy medicine and let thy medicine be thy food" – Hippocrates. We are what we eat, and it's one of the fastest ways to create change. Nutrients are our #3 cell and life fuel.

5. Ensure you're expelling toxins and your lymphatic system is operating efficiently – this is the waste disposal part of the immune system which works most efficiently when you're active. Consider yoga and rebounding! Get the heart rate and body temperature up a little. Expelling waste and toxins is the #4 'fuel' for our cells.

6. Meditate and gain an understanding of how your thoughts and emotions impact your biology. Chronic stress can compromise our health and immune system. Similarly, chronic thoughts of love and appreciation actually put your body into healing mode. Living in a state of appreciation and gratitude can strengthen your immune system and impact your biology in a positive way.

7. Find ways to release trauma and trapped emotions from the body. Trauma release exercises and yoga are an excellent place to start.

8. Make sure nothing in your mouth is compromising your electrical systems, namely mercury fillings, cavities and root canals. Seek a functional medicine doctor and/or bio-dentist and assess whether this is an area to address.

9. Read up! When you're ready, step into the field of quantum physics (don't let that sound like a scary term), and discover the healing ability beyond our physical bodies. This is when things get really, really, exciting.

10. Research people who have reversed what you're wishing to reverse. Seek solutions from those who have done it. Listen to *The Vitality Secret Podcast* in which I've interviewed people who have reversed 'incurable' illnesses, according to Western Medicine, read *The Vitality Secret,* and join my online program called 'Ignite Your Inner Healer.'

Neil Cannon - United Kingdom
Founder of Vitality Secret, Bestselling Author
www.VitalitySecret.com
◼ NeilCannon80
◎ NeilCannonVitality

The Ignite health and wellness authors set some intentions and
infused this Mandala - to support both writers and readers
in their health and wellness journey ....

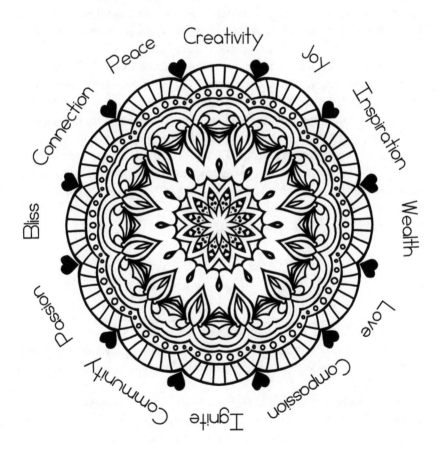

THANK YOU

Please know that every word written in this book, and every letter on the pages has been meticulously crafted with fondness, encouragement and a clarity to not just inspire you but to transform you. Many individuals in this book stepped up to share their stories for the very first time. They courageously revealed the many layers of themselves and exposed their weaknesses like few leaders do. Additionally, they spoke authentically from the heart and wrote what was true for them. We could have taken their stories and made them perfect, following every editing rule, but instead, we chose to leave their unique and honest voice intact. We overlooked exactness to foster individual expression. These are their words, their sentiments and explanations. We let their personalities shine in their writing so you would get the true sense of who each one of them is completely. That is what makes IGNITE so unique. Authors serving others, stories igniting humanity. No filters.

A tremendous thank you goes to those who are working in the background, editing, supporting, and encouraging the authors. They are some of the most genuine and heart-centered people I know. Their devotion to the vision of IGNITE, their integrity and the message they aspire to convey, is at the highest caliber possible. They too want you to find your IGNITE moment and flourish. They each believe in you and that's what makes them so outstanding. Their dream is for your dreams to come true.

Editing Team: Alex Blake, Andrea Drajewicz, Carmelita McGrath, Jock Mackenzie & Wendy Albrecht
Production Team: Dania Zafar, Peter Giesin & JB Owen

A special thanks and gratitude to the project leaders: Alex Jarvis and Annie Lebrun for their support behind the scenes and for going 'above and beyond' to make this a wonderful experience ensuring everything ran smoothly and with elegance.

A deep appreciation goes to each and every author who made Ignite your Health and Wellness possible — with all your heartfelt stories embracing this amazing idea of igniting others in their health and well being.

To all readers, we thank you for reading and loving the stories, for opening your hearts and minds to the idea of igniting your one lives. We welcome you to share your story and become a new author in one of our upcoming books. Sharing your message and Ignite moments be exactly what someone needs to hear.

Join us in the future on this magical 'Ignite' journey!

BOOKS AND RESOURCES MEANINGFUL TO THE IGNITE YOUR HEALTH AND WELLNESS AUTHORS

Alex Jarvis
https://en.wikipedia.org/wiki/Tzimtzum
https://www.britannica.com/topic/tzimtzum
http://www.walkingkabbalah.com/tsimtsum-tzimtzum/
https://www.chabad.org/library/article_cdo/aid/361884/jewish/Tzimtzum.htm

Annie Lebrun
www.bodymatrixspecialist.com

Brent McCord
Books:
- Undo it - Dean Ornish MD and Anne Ornish
- Mind over Medicine - Lissa Rankin MD
- Choose Yourself - James Altucher
- Love yourself like your life depends on it - Kamal Ravikant
- The Code of the Extraordinary Mind - Vishen Lakhiani

Videos:
- I am that I am - powerful affirmation based meditation by Dr. Wayne Dyer https://www.youtube.com/watch?v=A96OI4b8sFY
- 6 phase meditation - guided meditation by Vishen Lakhiani https://www.youtube.com/watch?v=oeQfRtiY-ZM&list=PLj0OeZJ7GZdAGShwEx-Vko1oxiYdV0X0MV&index=19

Charlene Ray
Devotions: The Selected Poems of Mary Oliver by Mary Oliver (Wild Geese poem)
What To Say When You Talk To Yourself by Shad Helmstetter, Ph.D
"Love After Love" is a poem by Derek Walcott, included in his Collected Poems, 1948–1984.

Claes Nermark
Overcoming Multiple Sclerosis, The evidence-based 7 step recovery program by Professor George Jelinec, MD

Dr. Gregory Damato
www.thesuperheroprogram.com

Hilde Jahren
www.getwildfit.com

Katarina Amadora
Grain Brain: The Surprising Truth about Wheat, Carbs, and Sugar--Your Brain's Silent Killers by David Perlmutter

LL Samantha Legassie
Hannasomatics.com, Hannasomatics.ca, Rejuvinagesomatics.ca
Somatics. Reawakening the minds control of movement, flexibility, and health by Dr Thomas Hanna

Marjan Tavakkolian
Www.maison38.com

Mystère Poème
Movies
  • Invisible Illness Film - http://InvisibleIllnessFilm.com/

Books
  • Ayurveda: The Science of Self-Healing by Dr. Vasant Lad
  • Prakriti: Your Ayurvedic Constitution by Dr. Robert E. Svoboda
  • Eat-Taste-Heal: An Ayurvedic Cookbook for Modern Living by Thomas Yarema and Daniel Rhoda

Healthcare Professional
  • Mary-Alice Quinn, AyD., C.A.S. Ayurvedic Doctor and Clinical Ayurvedic Specialist maryalicequinn.com

Wendy Albrecht
The Fifth Agreement book by Ruiz & Ruiz
What the Bleep Do We Know movie
Your intuition and emotions as life guides

Yaana Hauvroesh
Vision Quest Programs: Way of Nature - Sacred Passages with John Milton - https://www.healthpromoting.com/

Neil Cannon

True North Health Center - https://www.healthpromoting.com/
Tree of Life & Dr Gabriel Cousens - http://treeoflifecenterus.com/
Hippocrates Health Institute - https://hippocratesinst.org/
Ann Wigmore Natural Health Institute - https://annwigmore.org/
Earthing by Clinton Ober - https://grounded.com/
earthing-the-most-important-health-discovery-ever/earthing-book

PHOTO CREDITS

Upcoming Books in the
IGNITE SERIES
If you have story to share,
Please apply at www.igniteyou.life/apply

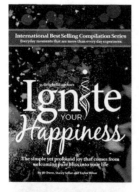

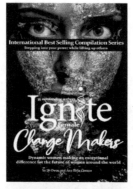

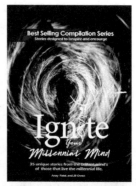

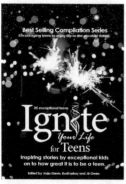

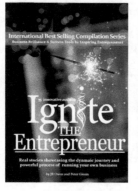

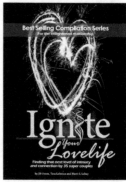

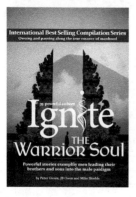

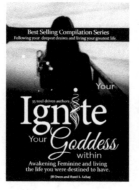

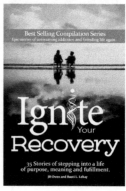